IMPROVING SKILLS

IN

SPEECH THERAPY

IMPROVING SKILLS
IN
SPEECH THERAPY

By

DORIS DAVIS WALLACE, Ph.D.
Formerly Assistant Professor of Speech
Supervisor of Speech Therapy
Northern Illinois University
De Kalb, Illinois

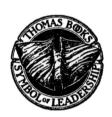

CHARLES C THOMAS · PUBLISHER
Springfield · Illinois · U.S.A.

Published and Distributed Throughout the World by
CHARLES C THOMAS • PUBLISHER
BANNERSTONE HOUSE
301-327 East Lawrence Avenue, Springfield, Illinois, U.S.A.
NATCHEZ PLANTATION HOUSE
735 North Atlantic Boulevard, Fort Lauderdale, Florida, U.S.A.

With THOMAS BOOKS *careful attention is given to all details of manufacturing and design. It is the Publisher's desire to present books that are satisfactory as to their physical qualities and artistic possibilities and appropriate for their particular use.* THOMAS BOOKS *will be true to those laws of quality that assure a good name and good will.*

Printed in the United States of America
W-1

PREFACE

THIS BOOK IS BASED on my experiences, which began thirteen years ago, as a supervisor of speech therapists. I have designed it to help the therapist make an effective transition from the theory of speech correction to the practice of speech therapy.

I have described some of my experiences with clients and therapists and have presented suggestions which are designed to help therapists improve their skills. Some of the descriptions suggest possible solutions to many of the basic problems of speech therapy; however, I do not intend for the book to be prescriptive. I hope, rather, that it will inspire the reader to evaluate himself to start the adventure of self-improvement and to find individual solutions to individual problems.

Students who have had the beginning courses in speech correction in preparation for careers in speech therapy, therapists who are practicing in public schools, clinics or hospitals, and pathologists who are teaching speech correction courses or are engaged in clinical research in colleges or universities are among those who may wish to read the book. Those pathologists who are teaching courses in clinical practice or public school methods may wish to use it as a text.

The improvement of skills in speech therapy would be easier if more information were available concerning the therapeutic process. The factors present in the skillful practice of speech therapy have not been determined and perhaps can never be fully determined. The titles of the chapters of the book indicate the skills that, in my opinion, are important in speech therapy. The titles are, in fact, the major divisions of a form that I have devised for evaluating the work of beginning therapists. These titles, as well as the content of the book, undoubtedly reflect my philosophy of the field and my approach to speech therapy which have been influenced by my professors at the University of Missouri, the State University of Iowa and New York University and by my colleagues, students and clients in Minnesota, New York, Nebraska and Illinois. It is apparent that I have been exposed to many points of view and the reader will discover that I have found much of value in each of them.

I am especially grateful to Doctors Louis Lerea, William Shearer and David Williams of Northern Illinois University for reading parts of the manuscript during various stages of the preparation.

The book will serve its purpose if it encourages the reader to reevaluate some of his ideas about, and his attitudes toward, himself, his clients and speech therapy.

DORIS D. WALLACE

CONTENTS

IMPROVING SKILLS

IN

SPEECH THERAPY

Chapter I

CLINICAL COMPETENCE

IN THIS CHAPTER the following subjects are discussed: the nature of clinical competence; beginning self-evaluation; increasing knowledge of phonetics, of the speech problem, of the client and of the learning process; and increasing basic skill.

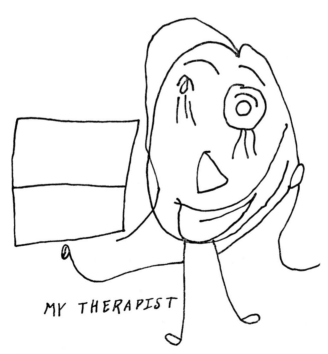

Drawn by an eight-year-old client who was attending an EMH class.

NATURE OF CLINICAL COMPETENCE

It has been estimated that from two to five per cent of all persons in the United States between five and twenty-one years of age have speech defects. Speech-defective individuals face many problems in a culture where oral communication is as important as it is in the United States, and they need the help of competent speech therapists.

It is difficult to define clinical competence in speech therapy. All of us agree that the competent therapist helps his clients improve their speech, but we are not sure what knowledge, understanding, attitudes and skills a therapist needs in order for improvement to take place. Few, if any, research studies have been completed that have related clinical competence to client improvement. The sparsity of research is no doubt due at least in part to: the difficulty of controlling factors other than clinical competence which affect client improvement; the lack of valid measures of clinical competence; and the lack of ability to control rater bias.

The following form for use in attempting to evaluate clinical competence was devised on the basis of the observation of more than one hundred therapy sessions. During each observation desirable and undesirable practices were described. The descriptions were then grouped and named.

Clinical Competence Form

Knowledge of:

1. Phonetics (aware of sounds in words, aware of the client's defective productions and understands the acceptable production of sounds);
2. The speech problem (understands the factors that are related to the problem and the currently accepted therapeutic procedures for it);
3. The client (is familiar with case history information, understands the client's feelings and the individual aspects of his problem);
4. The learning process (understands the importance of the client's involvement, moves from the simple to the more

complex after the simple is at least partially mastered, and considers the interest and ability level of the client).

Skill in:

1. Creating an atmosphere (is understanding, helpful and self-confident);
2. Using procedures (utilizes those that are related to the client's problem, focused and challenging);
3. Using methods and techniques (utilizes those that are related to the procedures, uses others after giving the first ones an adequate trial and explains them clearly);
4. Using materials and equipment (utilizes those that are sufficiently varied, original, adequately placed, and uses them fully);
5. Planning and reporting therapy sessions (writes prompt, professional and clear plans and reports—plans include an adequate number of activities which are related to the client's needs and which are designed to reduce difficulties during therapy sessions);
6. Evaluating therapy (is objective, has insight into own strengths and limitations, and desires to improve).

If the form has validity it is apparent that the competent speech therapist possesses extensive knowledge and is skilled in a variety of ways. Is it any wonder, then, that you who are beginning clinicians have some doubts and fears? You may question your ability to give the help your clients need, but you are also excited about the possibilities of using the procedures and methods you have studied. If you are an experienced therapist you may realize even more fully the complexity of your task and your limitations.

In order to increase your clinical competence it seems desirable that you follow the principle of learning through thinking and doing. This principle has been adhered to in this book by presenting descriptions of experiences therapists have had and by giving suggestions for improving knowledge and skill. Many more suggestions have been presented than you will be able to complete during one semester, but it is hoped that you will complete those that you believe will help you even after your clinical practice has been concluded.

Clinical competence is more, though, than the sum of your knowledge and skill. You should integrate these factors into a meaningful whole by applying knowledge of the field to clients in a skillful way.

BEGINNING SELF-EVALUATION

If you wish to increase your clinical competence you need to evaluate the present status of that competence. Other persons, including your supervisor, will help you discover your abilities and limitations, but careful self-evaluation is vital.

On the basis of the evaluation of approximately three hundred therapy sessions conducted in three different universities, beginning therapists rated high in knowledge of the client, skill in creating an atmosphere and skill in using materials and equipment, and they rated low in knowledge of phonetics. These therapists were familiar with data from the client's case history, they seemed to understand the client's feelings and the individual aspects of his problem. This knowledge probably helped them create a helpful, understanding atmosphere in which they usually appeared self-confident. They were skilled in using varied, somewhat original materials that were adequately placed and fully used, but they needed to improve their awareness of sounds in words, their awareness of the client's defecitve sound productions and their understanding of the acceptable production of sounds.

How do your abilities and limitations compare with those of these beginning therapists? If you wish to start self-evaluation, why not follow some of the following suggestions?

Suggestions for Beginning Self-evaluation

1. List some of your personal assets. How will they help you in your work as a speech therapist?

2. After reading some articles similar to the following, write a concise description of an effective speech therapist:

POWERS, M. H.: What makes an effective public school therapist? *J. Speech Hearing Dis., 21* (4) :461-467, Dec., 1956.

Speech Correctionists: The Competencies They Need for the Work They Do. Washington, D. C., U. S. Department of Health, Education and Welfare, Office of Education, Bulletin, 1957, No. 19.

HUDSON, M.: *Procedures for Teaching Trainable Children.* Washington, D. C., Council for Exceptional Children.

3. Tape-record one of your therapy sessions. As you listen to the recording, use the Clinical Competence Form presented in this chapter to help you decide what your abilities and limitations as a therapist are.

INCREASING KNOWLEDGE OF PHONETICS

Speech therapy, especially direct, phoneme-centered speech therapy often involves the teaching of phonetics. A therapist may sometimes find it necessary or desirable to teach the International Phonetic Alphabet, particularly when working with clients who have a foreign dialect; however, he will frequently teach clients to become aware of sounds in words, to become aware of defective sound productions and to produce sounds acceptably. If he does not posses these abilities himself, he will have difficulty teaching them to his clients.

Therapists we have observed often used drill words for articulation clients that revealed their lack of awareness of the sounds that combine to form a word. Some used words that did not contain the sound they were stressing in therapy; for example, "shoes" as a drill word for [tʃ], "houses" for [s], and "flowers" for [w]. Other therapists used "kite" with a client who was just beginning to improve his [t] for [k] substitution, "asleep" with a client who was beginning to improve his laterally emitted [s], and "this" with one who was beginning to improve his [θ] for [s] substitution. These words were, of course, very difficult for these clients.

Sometimes therapists labelled sounds in ways that confused their clients. For example, one said, "Today we will work on the 'sh' sound" to a client who was eight years of age and of average intelligence. When he tries to spell "Chicago" he will probably spell it with an "sh" if he articulates the word acceptably and if he has good auditory discrimination. Perhaps the therapist should have said, "Today we will learn to produce the [ʃ] sound," producing the sound itself. The client would have received auditory stimulation and been less confused about spelling. If the therapist had wanted to emphasize the development of spelling skills, he could have had the client think of words with different spellings that contain [ʃ]. Another therapist said, "Today we'll learn to make the 'c' sound." Did she mean [s], [z], [k], [ʃ] or [tʃ]?

Some therapists were not aware of their client's defective sound productions. They had particular difficulty discriminating [s] and [tʃ] from [ʃ], [s] from [z], [θ] from [ð], [d] from [ð], and [t] from [d]. Sometimes they did not hear the client insert his substituted sound between his production of the new sound and the vowel of a nonsense syllable or a word. Some therapists had difficulty hearing dentalized [t], [d], [tʃ] and [dʒ]. Others had as much difficulty hearing acceptable sound productions as defective ones and thus failed to build a list of key words that would have reduced the amount of time spent in therapy. Still others could not hear the minute differences in their clients' sound productions that indicated that they were improving.

Two therapists did not notice that in conversation their clients produced [b] with aspiration and that this was the reason their [b] resembled [p]. One was working with a client whose native language was Czech and the other with a client who was a severely hard-of-hearing young adult. The therapists wasted time by having these clients practice vibrating their vocal folds when they needed merely to produce [b] without aspiration.

The ability to hear unacceptable sound productions is especially important when recording the results of an articulation test. A knowledge of phonetics is also needed when analyzing the unacceptable productions. These aspects of therapy are discussed in Chapter II, "Using Diagnostic Tools."

Sometimes therapists who were giving direct, phoneme-centered therapy did not produce sounds in isolation in an acceptable manner and/or they did not remember how they are produce. Some therapists produced [θ], [ð], [f] and [v] in isolation as plosives rather than as continuants. Others had difficulty describing the acceptable production of [r], [ɝ], [ɚ] and [l]. Part of their difficulty was caused by their use of descriptive words that were not in their client's receptive vocabulary, but most of it seemed to be a result of an inability to remember the rather complicated process that is required for the production of these sounds.

Some therapists failed to remember that there are many acceptable methods of sound production and that the acoustic effect is of paramount importance. The cosmetic effect is not of paramount importance. The cosmetic effect is, of course, sometimes important. One therapist said that she did not realize that it was possible to produce an acceptable [s] using different placements of the tip of the tongue. Effective therapists noticed that a client was articulating some of his sounds with his teeth tightly clenched or with a low tongue position and helped him change these habits in order to improve the acoustic result. Some therapists forgot that the phonemes around the unacceptable one influence its production.

Are you aware of sounds in words? Are you aware of defective sound productions? Do you produce sounds acceptably? Can you describe acceptable sound production to your clients?

Suggestions for Increasing Knowledge of Phonetics

1. Use the International Phonetic Alphabet to transcribe a paragraph from a newspaper into the standard speech of your area.

2. Transcribe the first four sentences of each of the records of the Linguaphone Dialect Record Series. (Linguaphone Institute, 30 Rockefeller Plaza, New York 20, New York.)

3. Translate into American English transcribed passages from sources such as these:

FIELDS, V., AND BENDER, J.: *Voice and Diction,* New York, Macmillan, 1949.

MANSER, R., AND MULGRAVE, D.: *Conversations in Phonetic Transcriptions.* New York, Dutton, 1941.

Passages from *Rip Van Winkle.* Springfield, Merriam.

4. Take some of the self-checking tests and transcribe the abnormal speech passages from:

VAN RIPER, C., AND SMITH, D.: *An Introduction to General American Phonetics.* New York, Harper, 1962.

5. Tape-record nonsense syllables containing the sounds of American English. Later listen to the recording and transcribe them.

6. View films such as this one:

Articulatory Movements in the Production of English Speech Sounds. Washington, D. C., Central Office Film Library, Veterans Administration, Vermont Avenue and H. Street, N.W.

7. Explain the acceptable production of [r] to one of your university-aged clients who has difficulty with this sound after you study descriptions in books similar to these:

GRAY, G., AND WISE, C.: *The Bases of Speech.* New York, Harper, 1959.

THOMAS, C.: *Phonetics of American English.* New York, Ronald Press, 1958.

8. Construct a chart showing how five of the sounds that are difficult for your clients are produced. Label the divisions of the chart: vocal folds, lips, teeth, tongue, type of obstruction, etc. Include information from at least three books similar to these:

BRONSTEIN, A.: *The Pronunciation of American English.* New York, Appleton, 1960.

CARRELL, J., AND TIFFANY, W.: *Phonetics: Theory and Application to Speech Improvement.* New York, McGraw, 1960.

KENYON, J.: *American Pronunciation.* Ann Arbor, Wahr, 1951.

INCREASING KNOWLEDGE OF THE SPEECH PROBLEM

The primary purpose of many speech correction courses is to increase knowledge of speech problems. Students who have applied themselves diligently to the course work have a good foundation for speech therapy. The content of these courses is not repeated in this part of this chapter. Some examples of the application of knowledge are given. They are followed by some suggestions for increasing knowledge of speech problems.

It is important to understand the factors that are related to speech problems and the currently acceptable therapeutic procedures that are followed with clients who have the problems. Knowledge of related factors is applied when a diagnosis is made (see Chapter II, "Using Diagnostic Tools") and when therapy plans are written, especially the plan written at the beginning of the semester in which the semester's work is outlined (see Chapter VII, "Planning and Reporting Sessions"). The list of objectives and the proposed procedures reveal the therapist's knowledge of the client's speech problem (see Chapter VI, "Using Procedures").

A therapist who planned to use direct therapy with a client who was six years of age and whose unilateral incomplete cleft palate had been surgically repaired recently listed the following objectives in the semester plan:

1. Increase Ken's jaw, tongue and lip movement;
2. Improve his ability to discriminate vocal qualities;
3. Improve his phrasing and breath control;
4. Improve his articulation of [p], [b], [t] and [d] in syllables and phrases which contain many low front vowels.

Another therapist listed these objectives for a university-aged client whose hoarse voice problem was related to chronic laryngitis and vocal abuse. The client had been a cheerleader during her four years of high school. Voice therapy had been recommended by a laryngologist.

1. Improve Jean's ability to relax;
2. Encourage Jean to contact the University Counseling Service for help with her emotional problems;
3. Improve her ability to discriminate vocal qualities;
4. Shift the area of primary resonance from her throat to her mouth;
5. Decrease her loudness level and increase variations in pitch.

Both lists revealed that these therapists had an adequate knowledge of their client's problem, including some knowledge of recent research in cleft palate and voice.

Do you understand the factors that are related to, and the currently acceptable therapeutic procedures for the following speech problems?

Articulation problems
Voice problems

Cleft palate speech
Delayed speech and language
Aphasia
Speech of the cerebral palsied
Speech of the hard of hearing

Do you understand the various theoretical concepts of the etiology of stuttering? And the therapeutic procedures currently used with each concept?

Suggestions for Increasing Knowledge of the Problem

1. Evaluate articles on voice and articulation that are found in newspapers and popular magazines. Consult books similar to the following to help you with your evaluation:

BERRY, M., AND EISENSON, J.: *Speech Disorders.* New York, Appleton, 1956.

VAN RIPER, C., AND IRWIN, J.: *Voice and Articulation.* Englewood Cliffs, Prentice-Hall, 1958.

2. Construct an information sheet concerning delayed speech and language and/or speech of the hard-of-hearing for distribution to classroom teachers. Consult references similar to these:

DAVIS, H., AND SILVERMAN, S.: *Hearing and Deafness.* New York, Holt, 1960.

MYKLEHUST, H.: *Auditory Disorders in Children.* New York, Grune, 1954.

VAN RIPER, C.: *Speech Correction: Principles and Methods.* Englewood Cliffs, Prentice-Hall, 1963.

3. Review what you remember about aphasia or speech of the cerebral palsied. Supplement your knowledge by reading from sources similar to these:

BAKER, E.: An historical development of etiological concepts concerning aphasic speech and their influence upon aphasic speech rehabilitation. Ann Arbor, University Microfilms, 1954.

CRUICKSHANK, W., AND RAUS, G. (eds.): *Cerebral Palsy.* Syracuse, Syracuse U P, 1955.

GOLDSTEIN, K.: *Language and Language Disturbance.* New York, Grune, 1948.

PENFIELD, W., AND ROBERTS, L.: *Speech and Brain Mechanisms.* Princeton, Princeton U P, 1959.

TOWBIN, A.: *The Pathology of Cerebral Palsy.* Springfield, Thomas, 1961.

WEPMAN, J.: *Recovery From Aphasia.* New York, Ronald, 1951.

4. Make a study of some of the research related to cleft palate speech. Organize the material according to the following aspects—psychological, physical, physiological and phonetic. Consult sources similar to these:

Cleft Palate J., University of Missouri, Columbia, Missouri, American Cleft Palate Association, Charlotte G. Wells, Secretary.

HOLDSWORTH, W.: *Cleft Lip and Palate.* New York, Grune, 1951.

J Speech Hearing Res and J Speech Hearing Dis.

5. Listen to some of the tape-recorded lectures made by authorities in the field of speech pathology:

A Profile in Words of the Speech and Hearing Pathology Profession. Produced by Carl H. Scott, Hollywood, California, Magnetic Tape Duplicators.

Rehabilitation of the Adult Stutterer. 1312 W. Johnson Street, Madison, Wisconsin, Bureau of Audio-Visual Instruction. (Several tapes available.)

6. Increase your knowledge of the various theoretical concepts of the etiology of stuttering and the therapeutic procedures currently used with each concept by reading from references similar to these:

DIEHL, C.: *A Compendium of Research on Stuttering.* Springfield, Thomas, 1958.

EISENSON, J.: *Stuttering: A Symposium.* New York, Harper, 1958.

HAHN, E.: *Stuttering: Significant Theories and Therapies.* Stanford, Stanford U P, 1956.

JOHNSON, W.: *The Onset of Stuttering.* Minneapolis, U of Minn Press, 1958.

TRAVIS, L.: *Handbook of Speech Pathology.* New York, Appleton, 1957.

INCREASING KNOWLEDGE OF THE CLIENT

Therapists should be familiar with the client's case history, understand his behavior and some of his feelings, as well as his interests and the individual aspects of his problem.

At one time a person who was not trained in speech therapy was assigned to abstract information from clients' case histories.

He included much that was not useful in his abstracts, such as birth weight, the age at which a client learned to sit alone, etc., when these were within the normal limits. He could have just mentioned that the developmental history was normal. He sometimes wrote someone's opinion about a child as though it were a fact about the child, and often failed to include information that was essential to the planning of therapy, such as the child's approximate mental age. Sometimes he included incorrect information; for example, he said that one child was in the third grade. A careful inspection of the history revealed that the child had been in the third grade two years ago.

These facts and opinions taken from Carol's case history helped her therapist plan an effective therapy program for her:

Carol was seventeen years of age and until a month ago had lived in a small Iowa town with her father, stepmother and three younger half-sisters.

She was born with a complete bilateral cleft of the lip, hard and soft palates and had eleven surgical procedures to repair these structures. In April, 1963, she had a pharyngeal flap operation. She had frequent bilateral ear infections with some drainage which had been treated medically; however, her hearing acuity was within the normal limits.

She had direct speech therapy during her first eight years in school.

Carol's test results included:
127 IQ on an individual intelligence scale;
120 IQ on a picture vocabulary test;
95 percentile on a listening test;
"Well-adjusted" socially according to a test of personality;
Interested in scientific and clerical areas according to an occupational inventory;
No perceptual-motor dysfunction according to a memory for designs test;
Manometric readings were 5.8 with nose open and 9.4 with nose closed;
Hard palate was low vaulted and there was moderate movement of the lateral pharyngeal musculature according to the examiner who gave a peripheral speech mechanism examination.

Her present dormitory counselor expressed the opinion that Carol made many friends and exhibited "maturity." Her developmental reading teacher noted that she was attentive and had a great deal of initiative.

A therapist may increase his knowledge of the client not only by reading his case history but also by reading about children or adults who have similar problems. Jimmie, four years old, with delayed speech, often hurt other children physically. His clinician read a bulletin about children who hurt others and found that these children are often troubled, jealous, worried, anxious or frustrated. He asked his mother some questions and found that his mother believed that he resented the attention his grandmother was giving his cousin, John, who was also four years old. The therapist was able to help Jimmie with his problem by following the advice given by the author of the bulletin.

During one semester therapists worked with the following clients:

William, who was brain injured, sucked his thumb;

Tommy, who was hard of hearing, would not share materials;

Bobby, who was brain injured, wanted to run away;

Henry, who suffered from delayed speech, destroyed playground equipment;

Kate (seven years of age), who was hard of hearing, wet the bed;

Ted, who had an organic voice problem, was afraid to go to the Health Center;

Rodney, whose problem was delayed speech, drew pictures on the washroom wall and destroyed toys.

The therapists of these clients were encouraged to read about these behavior problems in order to help determine the factors related to the problems and to help the clients with them.

Ideally, before giving speech therapy to children, therapists should have many opportunities to observe and interact with both normal and exceptional children. One beginning therapist was assigned to Mary, a mentally retarded client. She believed that Mary exhibited many unusual behavior tendencies; however, actually Mary was rather typical of clients with similar intelligent quotients.

A therapist should try to understand some of his client's feelings. Therapists who work with cerebral palsied clients should remember that many of them have a fear of falling which is more than a physical fear, a fear of what others are going to do to them, a fear of being socially ostracized and a feeling of inferiority. Miss Jones worked with Ruth, a severely cerebral palsied girl of normal intelligence, seven years of age, who had just become a client in a residential program. Miss Jones helped Ruth write a letter to her mother and discovered more about Ruth's deep feelings that were interfering with therapy. Ruth wrote the following letter:

Dear Mom,

I want to go home. Come and get me. I am crying because I want to go home. It's no fun here. There is no one here like me. I can't do anything the others can. I will not eat if you leave me here. Please don't be mad at me, and please, please, please come and get me.

Love,
Ruth

It is also important to understand the client's interests and the individual aspects of his problem. One therapist believed that Jim, with an articulation problem, had few interests. She had difficulty engaging him in conversation because he did not seem interested in anything. She had him check the play activities that he participated in on a list of such activities, and found that he was interested in crossword puzzles, boating, collecting butterflies and playing football. She was able to plan therapy sessions around some of these interests.

Another therapist who was working with an adult "expressive" aphasic client listed the following aspects of his problem, several of which were typical of other "expressive" aphasic clients:

Mark recently read Sandberg's three-volume work on Abraham Lincoln.

When he couldn't remember a word, he said "no, no" or used a synonym.

He had difficulty using many of the common prepositions. Most of his responses consisted of single words.

He used a high vocal pitch, a fast rate and a loud volume, especially when talking with strangers. He had difficulty articulating [t], [p] and [b] in the initial position.

His writing paper needed to be triple-spaced and he wrote best when he used a bowling scoring pencil wrapped in clay. He was able to write only two or three sentences before becoming exhausted.

Miss Smith, who was working with a university-aged client who stuttered, included the following scores and evaluations in her initial therapy plan:

Score	Test or Form	Evaluation
2.51	An attitude toward stuttering scale.	Jim had a considerable intolerance of stuttering.
10 minutes per day	Speaking time record.	Jim spoke less than the average adult
9.8%	Frequency of stuttering.	Jim was a moderate to severe stutterer.
39.7%	Consistency of stuttering.	His stuttering was less consistent than the average stutter's.
0%	Adaptation of stuttering.	He adapted much less than the average stutterer.

She also noticed that Jim's secondary symptoms included dilating his nostrils and moving his articulators in a silent attempt to form the initial sound of the word on which he was blocking.

Are you familiar with your client's case history? Do you understand some of his behavior and feelings? And are you acquainted with his interests and the individual aspects of his problem?

Suggestions for Increasing Knowledge of the Client

1. Present the complete case history and current status of your client to a group of colleagues.

2. Read about the behavior problems of children who have problems similar to those of your clients in sources like this one: RIDENOUR, N., AND JOHNSON, I.: *Some Special Problems of Children, Aged 2 to 5 Years.* 10 Columbus Circle, New York, The National Association for Mental Health, Inc., 1947.

3. Simulate the defect of your client in several situations. Analyze what you learned about your client from this experience.

4. Have one of your older clients check his interests on the list of play activities given on page 208 in:

WITTY, P.: *Reading in Modern Education.* Boston, Heath, 1949.

5. Obtain additional information about the speech behavior of one of your university-aged clients who stutters by following some of the procedures in:

JOHNSON, W., and others: *Diagnostic Methods in Speech Correction.* New York, Harper, 1962.

INCREASING KNOWLEDGE OF THE LEARNING PROCESS

In this part of this chapter some general principles of learning, with examples taken primarily from direct phoneme-centered therapy sessions with university-aged clients illustrating the principles, and suggestions for increasing knowledge of the learning process are presented.

There is some research to substantiate the point of view that the therapist should understand the importance of the client's involvement in the therapy session. Active participation by the client is preferable to passive reception. The type of involvement is determined, in part, at least, by the approach the therapist uses. (See Chapter III, "Creating an Atmosphere.")

In direct phoneme-centered therapy, especially with older clients, the therapy should be dominated by a purpose which the client has set. The client needs practice in setting realistic goals which are challenging, but which yield some success. Sometimes the therapist fails not only to have the client set the goal, but also to inform the client of the purpose that the therapist has set. One university-aged client complained to a friend that she did not know what she was doing in therapy or why she was doing it.

Often the therapist evaluates all of the client's sound productions. During many therapy sessions the client looked hopefully at the therapist after every attempt at sound production. Either ear training had not been successful or the therapist was not taking advantage of the skill the client had acquired.

The therapist should move from what is simple for the particular client to what is more complex after the simple is at least partially mastered. There seems to be no substitute for practice in learning to speak more acceptably.

One therapist who was using direct therapy with a university-aged client with an articulation problem had him attempt to produce [k] in words before he had mastered its production in nonsense syllables. Another therapist used words containing [sts] with a client who had difficulty producing an acceptable [s] in almost all contexts. A third therapist continued to have a client repeat words containing [r] in the initial position when he produced every word with [w]. He seemed to be practicing his substitution.

Sometimes therapists did not move to more complex activities after the more simple ones had been mastered. One therapist did not introduce another sound after [d] had been mastered in conversational speech. Other therapists continued ear training exercises with clients who had normal hearing after they had frequently produced the sound being stressed in the ear training.

The therapist should consider the interest and ability level of the client and should attempt to create a constructive emotional climate. (See Chapter III, "Creating an Atmosphere.")

One therapist had difficulty working with Thelma, a severely cerebral palsied client, seven years of age, with very few interests and a mental age of approximately two years, six months. The therapist was encouraged to make the therapy sessions more enjoyable for Thelma. She discovered that Thelma enjoyed rolling a ball, clapping to the rhythm of phonograph records, hitting the keys of a piano, turning the light "on" and "off," and opening and closing the door. She also enjoyed talking over a toy telephone, treating the therapist like a doll by brushing her hair and buttoning and unbuttoning her jacket.

Sometimes a therapist needs to consider one aspect of the learning process and decide how he may improve this aspect. One day a therapist who was working with adolescent clients read a sentence in a text that encouraged him to consider how he was using praise. The author of the text pointed out that the consequences of an action should be presented without praise or blame. He realized that he had been using praise quite liberally. He decided that before he stopped using it he would consult other texts. He found that behaviorists and other theorists do not agree with regard to praise. He reasoned that he was adding to his clients' instability by treating them like adults in that he was encouraging them to assume responsibility for improving their own speech and was trying to create a permissive atmosphere; but he was treating them like children in that they may have been dependent upon his praise. He decided that he would vary the amount of praise he used. In beginning therapy sessions when the sessions were more therapist-controlled he would use more praise, and as the sessions continued and became more client-centered he would decrease the amount of praise. He decided that in beginning sessions the clients probably needed to realize that they counted and that someone knew they were there; however, he did try to become more skilled in communicating these feelings without the use of praise. He also decided that he would vary the amount of praise according to the emotional age of the client.

Do you understand the basic principles of learning? Are you acquainted with some of the theories of learning? And are you able to apply what you know about learning?

Suggestions to Increase Knowledge of the Learning Process

1. Recall some of the principles used by the best teachers you had in elementary school after reading some of the chapters from:

PETERSON, H. (ed.): *Great Teachers*: *Portrayed by Those Who Studied Under Them*. Rutgers, 1946.

2. Read about a theory of learning that is new to you and apply it when writing your next week's therapy plan. Evaluate the results. Consult references, such as:

CANTOR, N.: *The Dynamics of Learning*. Buffalo, Foster and Stewart, 1946.

MATIS, M.: The application of modern theories of learning to speech therapy. *Western Speech*, 15:44-48.

MOWRER, O. H.: *Learning Theory and Personality Dynamics*. New York, Ronald, 1950.

3. Compare several theories of learning on one aspect of the problem and formulate your own conclusions. Consult references

such as these:

ESTES, W. K., and others: *Modern Learning Theory*. New York, Appleton, 1954.

HILGARD, E. R.: *Theories of Learning*. New York, Appleton, 1956.

SMITH, H. P.: *Psychology in Teaching*. Englewood Cliffs, Prentice-Hall, 1954.

INCREASING BASIC SKILL

There are certain activities a therapist can engage in that will increase his knowledge of speech correction and improve many of the skills he needs when working with speech defective individuals. Some of the activities are: attending meetings; observing other therapists; and working with clients under supervision. Some therapists, of course, need to enroll for additional courses in speech correction and/or related fields.

Attending national conventions of the American Speech and Hearing Association improves clinical competence. The following titles of some of the papers presented at two recent conventions indicate the variety of programs presented and suggest some of the benefits to be derived from attendance:

"Cleft Palate Speech: Implications from Research for Diagnosis and Therapy";

"Personality Characteristics of Veterans with Hearing Losses";

"The Role of Reinforcement in First Language Learning";

"Testing Children with Multiple Handicaps";

"Client-Clinician Relationships and Concomitant Factors in Stuttering Therapy";

"The Relationship of Auditory Discrimination to Language Learning";

"Techniques of Teaching the [r] Sound";

"An Automated Speech Correction Program";

"Records and Reports for Public School Speech and Hearing Programs."

At one of these conventions two of the short courses offered were "Language Problems in Children" and "Emotional Problems of the Cleft Palate Child." The stimulation and information received in informal conversations at conventions is also, of course, important.

Regional and local organizations have informative meetings. At one recent regional meeting, "Voice Problems of Children" were discussed and clients were presented. Therapists in some school systems meet frequently for presentation of papers on research studies and presentation of their more difficult clients.

Another effective method for improving basic skill is to observe therapists with different training backgrounds working in a variety of settings. During one semester student therapists observed sessions in a suburban public school, a city public school, a veterans' hospital, a city hospital, a private speech and hearing clinic, a children's hospital and a university speech clinic.

Probably one of the best procedures for increasing basic skill is to work with clients under supervision. The following are statements therapists wrote in answer to the question, "What have you learned this semester by working with out-patient clients?"

My clients have helped me put into practice the theories of therapy that I studied in other classes.

Speech correction is the field for me, for it has given me many satisfying rewards.

I have learned the importance of adequate diagnosis.

Sound substitutions are often embedded in a client's speech behavior.

One type of therapy will help one client but not another.

A client's attitude toward therapy is very important.

I have gained insight into the problems and personality of an aphasic client.

I had an apathetic client who forced me to become imaginative and resourceful.

Working with clients has increased my self-confidence.

I have learned to be more patient.

The methods used in therapy should be simple enough for the client to follow easily.

Effective therapy requires thoughtful planning.

When asking a question, it is important not to suggest

the answer.

I now know what my weak areas are, and I am finding ways to improve.

Suggestions for Increasing Basic Skill

1. Discuss at one of your group meetings some of the questions given in:

VAN RIPER, C.: *A Case Book in Speech Therapy.* Englewood Cliffs, Prentice-Hall.

2. Observe some therapy sessions and compare what you observe with the practices suggested in references similar to the following:

BERRY, M., AND EISENSON, J.: *Speech Disorders.* New York, Appleton, 1956.

JOHNSON, W., and others: *Speech Handicapped School Children.* New York, Harper, 1956.

VAN RIPER, C. (ed.): *Speech Therapy: A Book of Readings.* Englewood Cliffs, Prentice-Hall, 1953.

Chapter II

USING DIAGNOSTIC TOOLS

As you may have noticed, "using diagnostic tools" does not appear on the Clinical Competence Form presented in Chapter I. The form was used to evaluate the work of therapists who were not making major diagnostic decisions. It seems desirable, however, to improve ability to use diagnostic tools and to use the information obtained to improve therapy. The present chapter includes a discussion of diagnostic tools and presents suggestions for improving skill in using these tools.

SCREENING EVALUATIONS

The ability to understand and use American English varies from one individual to another. The following descriptions concern clients who had severe speech and/or language defects:

A seven-year-old boy whose many sound substitutions, additions and omissions made it impossible to tell which nursery rhyme he was repeating;

An adult male who had to use an electrolarynx;

A university-aged stutterer whose average rate of speaking was ten words per minute;

A five-year-old girl with a severe hearing loss who did not understand the meaning of simple words such as boy, baby and hello;

An eight-year-old mongoloid who replied "that's lovely" or "wonderful" to almost every remark that was made to her;

An elderly expressive aphasic who made his wants known by writing notes.

Other individuals are skilled speakers who often make their living by talking. They may include actors, politicians, lawyers and teachers.

During a process called screening, a therapist decides whether or not an individual has acceptable speech. The individual may belong to a group in which each member is having his speech evaluated. One of the difficult decisions the therapist makes during screening concerns the individual who has a relatively minor speech difference.

A therapist who was screening the freshman class of a college included in her case load many clients with hypernasal voices. As the screening continued, she discovered that many students possessed this quality and she decided that she could not include all of them in her case load. She realized, though, that some would eventually move from the region; therefore, she decided not to rely entirely upon the norms of the group. Perhaps she should have asked the individuals whether or not they wanted speech therapy. In many settings, individuals, even those with severe defects, or their parents make the decision.

You may choose the type or types of screening evaluations you use from among those that are similar to those listed in Suggestion Two at the close of the chapter. You may wish to use some of them at the beginning of a regular diagnostic session or toward the beginning of a period of therapy in order to make valid decisions concerning the additional evaluations that are needed.

Factors other than the differences that exist between a prospective client's speech and the speech of his peers are sometimes important in determining who needs therapy. His attitude toward his difference, the attitudes of his friends and relatives and the amount of talking he will do in his chosen occupation are factors that probably should be considered.

Some therapists are disturbed when a client whom they would not choose is included in a case load. It is important to realize that this value judgment varies even when made by experienced, well-trained therapists. Sometimes, too, the decision is determined by practical considerations. For instance, a therapist may include clients with minor differences when her case load is small.

After a therapist has decided that an individual needs speech therapy, she makes several evaluations of his speech and language abilities. The evaluations should probably not be made until after a helping relationship has been established, unless such a relationship can be established during the testing. In some settings it is impossible to give all of the clients additional evaluations.

EVALUATION OF SPEECH AND LANGUAGE ABILITIES

Sometimes, beginning therapists, especially those who have not taken courses in diagnostics, are not aware of the many evaluations that they may make of the speech and language abilities of clients. The number and kind of evaluations made are related, of course, to the type of defect the client seems to possess and to certain characteristics of the client. It seems desirable, however, to describe as completely as possible the client's abilities toward the beginning of a period of therapy and to continue evaluation throughout therapy. Most of the evaluations that a therapist makes help improve therapy. It seems desirable, therefore, to make too many evaluations rather than too few.

Several types of evaluations are listed in Suggestion Three at the close of the chapter. Evaluations of a client's hearing are not included because they are beyond the scope of the book.

You may wish to consider questions similar to these when deciding which evaluations to make:

> What is known about the client's ability to articulate the sounds of American English? to use his voice? to understand speech? to formulate and express his thoughts?
>
> What do you need to know about these abilities in order to plan therapy for this semester?
>
> Which evaluations will help you discover more concerning what you need to know?

Perhaps your supervisor will assist you in evaluating your tentative answers to these questions. He may also indicate which evaluations you are not qualified to make.

EVALUATION OF RELATED FACTORS

Ideally, professionally trained personnel from many fields should work as a team to study the factors that may be related to a client's speech and/or language defect. Often, however, the therapist is responsible for studying the client and his history. She will, of course, refer a client who seems to have relatively severe problems in specific areas to the proper respresentative of the appropriate specialty.

One semester, four clients who had been born with cleft palates were enrolled in a clinic for therapy. Not only did the speech and language of the clients vary greatly but also the related factors that were studied. The following brief descriptions, based upon a considerable amount of evidence, suggest how varied the problems were:

Cathy (eight years old)
    Superior marks in school.
    Possible over protection by parents;
    Below-average social adjustment.

Bill (seven years old)
    Severe high-frequency bilateral hearing loss;
    Mother had a repaired cleft palate, inferior articulation and hypernasality;
    Low socioeconomic class;
    Possible parental hostility.

Grace (nine years old)
    IQ—73 on Peabody Vocabulary Test, Form A;
    Native language—Spanish;
    Below-average marks in school.

Glenn (seven years old)
    Short attention span;
    Hyperactive;
    Below-average auditory memory span;
    Unpredictable behavior.

The importance of investigating related factors is also illustrated by some of the difficulties a university-aged client had experienced. At the time she enrolled for therapy she stated that she had had speech therapy for as long as she could remember; that her parents often commented unfavorably about her lack of ability to participate in sports and that during her teens some of her acquaintances laughed at the way she walked. At the time of the initial interview, the therapist noticed that she talked out of the left side of her mouth, had difficulty raising her tongue-tip and distorted her sibilants. She was referred to the college physician, who referred her to a neurologist. His report stated that she had mild cerebral palsy. After a brief period of speech therapy, she was dismissed because it became evident that she had improved her speech as much as she was capable of improving it. The therapist believed that the client's elementary school therapy would have been more effective and her life happier if her physical difference had been diagnosed in her early childhood.

Several types of evaluations of the factors that may be related to a client's speech and/or language defect are listed in Suggestion Seven at the close of the chapter. Before deciding whether or not you wish to use a particular evaluation, you may wish to obtain some information about it, including some of the following:

Type of test (for example, a classification or a diagnostic test);
Purpose of the test and the subtests;
Theoretical basis;
Type and age of suitable clients;
Reliability;
Validity;
Methods of standardization;
Administration conditions, including qualification of examiner, instructions for administration, recording responses, time limits, etc.

SUMMARY OF EVALUATIONS

Before deciding upon a tentative diagnosis, or whether or not referrals should be made and/or what type of therapy to try, you should summarize the findings of your evaluations.

Sources of forms that you may use are listed in Suggestion Eight at the close of the chapter.

The following summary of evaluations was written at the conclusion of diagnostic sessions that were conducted by a speech pathologist, an audiologist, a pediatrician, a neurologist, a social worker and a school psychologist. The recommendations illustate how diagnostic information may contribute to the planning of therapy. Identifying material has been removed.

Speech and Language Abilities

The examiner talked with Bobby briefly and then administered the Templin-Darley screening test of articulation. Bobby distorted the following phonemes in at least one position: [l], [s], [z], [ʃ] and [tʃ]. He substituted other phonemes for these phonemes in at least one position: [y], [d], [f], [v], [θ], [ʒ], [j] and [tʃ]. He omitted these phonemes in at least one position: [θ], [ð] and [w]. The following phonemes were not articulated correctly during the test or following stimulation: [s], [z] and [tʃ]. He had more difficulty with the middle position in the word than with other positions and he frequently substituted a plosive for a fricative. He experienced no difficulty in using voiced or voiceless phonemes and usually produced a phoneme with proper general placement of his articulators. His speech was intelligible when the listener knew the topic of conversation. His voice quality was within the normal limits for a child of his age and sex.

On May 28, 1965, when Bobby was eight years and seven months old, the Illinois Test of Psycholingiustic Abilities was administered. His language ages on the subtests were as follows:

Auditory-Vocal Automatic	5-9
Visual Decoding	6-8
Motor Encoding	above the norms
Auditory-Vocal Association	6-6
Visual-Motor Sequencing	8-5
Vocal Encoding	3-6
Auditory-Vocal Sequencing	5-11
Visual-Motor Association	8-11
Auditory Decoding	8-10

These results indicate that Bobby had particular difficulty using grammar, describing simple objects and remembering digits. His total score language age on the test was 6-10.

Related Factors

Bobby's parents first regarded him as having defective speech when he was three years old. At this time the only word in his vocabulary was no. His mother stated that he frequently got by without using speech, that he was a very quiet baby, drooled excessively and was bottle-fed. She also reported great difficulty in getting him to take food and in toilet training.

His mother's health during pregnancy was good, labor lasted approximately three hours and delivery was normal; however, he was hospitalized for two weeks after birth with an elevated temperature and jaundice. His mother had Rh negative and his father Rh positive bood types.

Pure tone audiometric air conduction testing with a Beltone 10C audiometer indicated hearing was within the normal limits bilaterally. Bobby had difficulty discriminating sounds, especially those he misarticulated. He also had difficulty synthesizing sounds into words. His auditory memory span for consonants was greatly below average, while his memory span for vowels was somewhat below average.

His extremities were hypertonic and became stiff when he was approached. Patellar reflexes were not obtained and Babinski was absent. He walked with an unsteady spastic gait and performed the finger-nose test unsteadily. The electroencephalographic record showed bursts of paroxysmal high voltage and slow activity which was believed to indicate deep-lying dysfunction.

An examination of the speech mechanism revealed that lip mobility was adequate for purposes of speech production, although protrusion was poor and extraneous movement was noticed. Bobby protruded his tongue adequately, but he was unable to touch the corners of his mouth with his tongue. His hard palate was normal in height and in cuspid and molar width. His soft palate functioned adequately.

On the performance scale of the Wechsler Intelligence Scale for Children, Bobby's intelligence quotient was 93. He had difficulty with the puzzle test. On the Arthur Point Scale, his intelligence quotient was 95 and he was particularly low

in abstract thinking. On the Bender Gestalt Test, his performance seemed typical of a brain-damaged child.

On the Vineland Scale of Social Maturity, Bobby scored a
social age of eight years six months; however, the examiner
believed that his mother answered the questions in such a way
as to create a good impression of Bobby's abilities. Bobby's
mother was a registered nurse before her marriage and his
father was department supervisor in a local factory at the
time of the interview. Members of the family were close. They
liked to play games together, go on picnics and do other things
together. Bobby's siblings were a brother and a sister twelve
and eleven years old. Apparently Bobby's family understood
and accepted his difference, and according to the social worker
there was little evidence of emotional problems. Bobby
appeared shy and was reluctant to talk during the interview,
but he seemed to relate well to the examiners. His mother
reported that he got along well with his friends; however, they
were younger than he.

DIAGNOSIS: Moderately severe articulation and severe
language defect related to cerebral palsy of a mixed type and
possible aphasia. (The medical specialists made the diagnosis
of cerebral palsy and possible aphasia.)

PROGNOSIS: Guarded.

RECOMMENDATIONS: Intensive speech and language therapy
presented after a helping relationship has been established,
using structured therapy sessions, but with one of the primary
objectives to make communication enjoyable and profitable.
Other objectives may be chosen from some similar to the
following:

1. To improve ability to discriminate between plosives and
fricative sounds, especially those misarticulated;

2. To improve ability to discriminate between acceptable
and unacceptable consonant production in the medial
position of words frequently used;

3. To improve auditory memory span, especially for complete words;

4. To improve ability to synthetize sounds into words;

5. To improve movement of articulators, especially the
tongue;

6. To improve articulation of consonant sounds, starting

with the [l], [v] and [ð], stressing visual, kinesthetic and
tactile stimuli. Use auditory stimuli if the auditory training
is partially successful;
7. To improve ability to use the grammar of American
English, especially the use of adjectives;
8. To increase the mean length of response.

When a therapist works in a setting where she cannot consult
other specialists, it sometimes seems desirable to defer the making
of referrals, especially those to specialists who study emotional
and behavioral problems.

One winter day eight-year-old Lucy, accompanied by her
mother, came to the Clinic for a speech evaluation. Lucy was
diagnosed as having severely retarded speech and language.
The examiner believed that Lucy should be referred for
psychological evaluations because she was reluctant to talk,
she and her mother seemed depressed, and her mother stated
that Lucy cried every night when her father attempted to
help her with homework. In fact, Lucy's mother criticized
many aspects of her husband's behavior, especially his discipline practices. The examiner, however, decided to have
them return in two weeks. When they returned they both
seemed happier. Lucy's mother explained that the steel strike
had been settled and that her husband and son had returned
to work. During the first interview, she had labelled her
husband's occupation in such a way that the examiner had not
been aware that he was on strike. The examiner decided to
recommend a conference between the father and the public
school therapist and observe Lucy's behavior during therapy
sessions for possible indications of related emotional factors.

Sam, a nine-year-old severe stutterer, had seemed fairly
well adjusted during the initial diagnostic session. During
therapy sessions, however, his behavior led the therapist to
recommend testing at a local mental health clinic where
parental referral was accepted. His conversation often con-
concerned guns and killing and when the war comes with
Russia. During one therapy session, he drew a picture of his
older brother walking on crutches, with cuts on his face and
two black eyes. Sam explained, "This is the way he'll look
when he gets out of the hospital after I beat him up." On

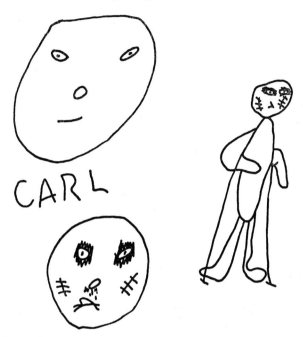

Pictures drawn by a nine-year-old stutterer of his brother, showing him before he went to the hospital and after he came from the hospital following a beating that the client wanted to give him.

Rogers' Personality Adjustment Inventory, Sam made high scores on "Personal Inferiority," "Family Maladjustment" and "Day Dreaming." Some of his responses were, "I want my father and mother to love me," "They always treat my brother better than me," and "I don't like my brothers and sisters—I don't like them at all."

If you wish to improve certain aspects of your ability to evaluate speech and language and the factors that may be related to clients' defects, follow some of these suggestions:

Suggestions for Improving Skill in Using Diagnostic Tools

1. Increase your knowledge concerning diagnosis in speech correction by reading from references similar to these:

DARLEY, F.: *Diagnosis and Appraisal of Communication Disorders.* Englewood Cliffs, Prentice-Hall, 1964.

MYKLEBUST, H.: *Auditory Disorders in Children.* New York, Grune, 1954.

TRAVIS, L. (ed.): *Handbook of Speech Pathology.* New York, Appleton, 1957. Consult chapters written by Bloomer, Eisenson, Goodhill, Koepp-Baker, Milisen, Moore, Myklebust, Powers, and Steer and Hanley.

2. Administer some of the following screening evaluations to at least four prospective clients. (Several sources of the same type of evaluation are listed because some of the sources may not be readily available to you. If the evaluation is found in a book, the name of the authors, book and publishers are given the first time the source is mentioned. Additional listings include only the authors' names.)

CONVERSATIONAL SPEECH

Elicit conversational speech by asking questions. Consult:

JOHNSON, W., DARLEY, F., AND SPRIESTERBACH, D.: *Diagnostic Methods in Speech Pathology.* New York, Harper, pp. 204-206. Milisen in Travis, p. 287.

RECITATION OF LEARNED MATERIAL

Clients may count, recite the pledge of allegiance to the flag, nursery rhymes, etc.

ORAL READING OF PARAGRAPHS

ANDERSON, V.: *Improving the Child's Speech.* New York, Oxford U P, 1953, pp. 51-52.

————: *Training the Speaking Voice.* New York, Oxford U P, 1961, pp. 17-21.

FAIRBANKS, G.: *Voice and Articulation Drillbook.* New York, Harper, 1960, p. 127.

IRWIN, R.: *Speech and Hearing Therapy.* Englewood Cliffs, Prentice-Hall, 1953, p. 32.

JOHNSON, DARLEY, AND SPRIESTERSBACH, *op. cit.*, p. 233.

VAN RIPER, C.: *Speech Correction: Principles and Methods.* Englewood Cliffs, Prentice-Hall, 1963, p. 484.

ORAL READING OF SENTENCES

ANDERSON (1953), *op. cit.*, p. 58.

FAIRBANKS, *op. cit.*, pp. xiii-xvii.

IRWIN, *op. cit.*, p. 33.

SCHOOLFIELD, L.: *Better Speech and Better Reading.* Magnolia, *Expression*, 1951, pp. 2-5.

WEST, R., ANSBERRY, M., AND CARR, A.: *The Rehabilitation of Speech.* New York, Harper, 1957, p. 666.

SHORT ARTICULATION TEST

The clients may name objects or pictures found in the following:

ANDERSON (1953), *op. cit.*, pp. 53-57.

Bryngelson-Glaspey Speech Improvement Cards. Chicago, Scott, 1941.

IRWIN, *op. cit.*, pp. 31-32.

Templin-Darley Tests of Articulation. Iowa City, Bureau of Educational Research and Services, State University of Iowa. (Nondiagnostic items.)

The clients may read word lists or repeat them after the therapist, as found in:

IRWIN, *op. cit.*, p. 33.

The clients may repeat nonsense syllables, sounds in isolation or nonsense words, as found in:

Ibid., p. 77.

VAN RIPER, *op. cit.*, p. 229.

LANGUAGE SCREENING TEST

BARRY, H.: *The Young Aphasic Child.* Washington, D. C., The Volta Bureau, 1961, pp. 7-8.

AMMONS, R., AND AMMONS, H.: *Quick Vocabulary Test.* Missoula, Montana, Psychological Test Specialists, Box 1441, 1962.

EISENSON, J.: *Examining for Aphasia.* New York, Psychological Corporation, 1954. (Initial item of each subtest.)

WEPMAN, J., AND JONES, L.: *The Language Modalities Test for Aphasia.* Chicago, Education Industry Service, 1961. (Initial items.)

You may evaluate the speech samples as you obtain them or as you listen to tape recordings of the samples, by using forms similar to those found in these sources:

ANDERSON (1961), *op. cit.*, pp. 15-16.

CYPREANSEN, L., WILEY, J., AND LAASE, L.: *Speech Development, Improvement and Correction.* New York, Ronald, 1959, pp. 146-147.

FAIRBANKS, *op. cit.*, p. x.

JOHNSON, DARLEY, AND SPRIESTERSBACH, *op. cit.*, pp. 78-79.

Powers in Travis, p. 772.

3. Analyze the speech and language of a client by administering appropriate evaluations. Sometimes an appropriate evalu-

ation for a particular client may be listed under a type of evaluation other than the one you would expect to administer. For instance, a client with primarily a voice problem may be administered some of the evaluations listed under "Stuttering." Obtain the evaluations from sources similar to these:

Evaluation of Articulation

STRUCTURED ACTIVITY

VAN RIPER, C., AND IRWIN, J.: *Voice and Articulation.* Englewood Cliffs, Prentice-Hall, 1958, p. 59.

NAMING OBJECTS

The therapist may collect objects after consulting the following:

IRWIN, *op. cit.,* p. 79.

WEST, ANSBERRY, AND CARR, *op. cit.,* pp. 670-671.

The therapist may purchase the following:

FERGEN AND WILLIAMS: *Fer-Will Object Kit.* The King Company, 4906 North Tripp Avenue, Chicago 30, Illinois.

THERAPIST CONSTRUCTED PICTURE TEST

IRWIN, *op. cit.,* pp. 77-79.

JOHNSON, DARLEY, AND SPRIESTERSBACH, *op. cit.,* pp. 86-89.

VAN RIPER, *op. cit.,* p. 230 and p. 482.

WEST, ANSBERRY, AND CARR, *op. cit.,* pp. 670-671.

PURCHASED PICTURE TEST

BARKER, J.: *The Arizona Articulation Proficiency Scale.* 12035 Wilshire Boulevard, Los Angeles, California, Western Psychological Services.

CLARK, R.: *Picture Phonetic Inventory.* Box 8865, University Park Station, Denver, Communication Foundation, Ltd.

EDMONSTON, W.: *The Laradon Articulation Scale.* Denver, Laradon Hall, 1960.

HEJNA, R.: *Developmental Articulation Test.* Box 1713, Ann Arbor, Michigan, Speech Materials.

MONTGOMERY, J.: *Look and Say Articulation Test.* 4906 North Tripp Avenue, Chicago 30, Illinois, The King Company.

Picture books that may be used as tests:

McCAUSLAND, M.: *Speech Through Pictures.* Magnolia, Expression, 1947.

STODDARD, C.: *Sounds for Little Folks.* Magnolia, Expression, 1940.

Pictures in speech correction texts:

ANDERSON (1953), *op. cit.*, pp. 53-57.

CYPREANSEN, WILEY, AND LAASE, *op. cit.*, pp. 149-164.

SPEECH TESTING FILMSTRIP

CYPREANSEN, L.: *Speech Testing Filmstrip*. Lincoln, University of Nebraska, Speech and Hearing Laboratories.

WORD LIST

FAIRBANKS, *op. cit.*, pp. 27-101.

MILISEN IN TRAVIS, *op. cit.*, pp. 286-287.

WEST, ANSBERRY, AND CARR, *op. cit.*, pp. 669-670.

LIST OF SENTENCES

ANDERSON (1953), *op. cit.*, pp. 58-59.

CYPREANSEN, WILEY, AND LAASE, *op. cit.*, pp. 164-171.

FAIRBANKS, *op. cit.*, pp. 27-101.

LAASE, L.: *Speech Project and Drill Book*. Dubuque, Brown, W C, pp. 204-206.

VAN RIPER, *op. cit.*, p. 483.

WEST, ANSBERRY, AND CARR, *op. cit.*, pp. 667-668.

INTELLIGIBILITY TEST

BLACK, J.: Danville, Illinois, The Interstate Publishers.

STIMULABILITY TEST

MILISEN IN TRAVIS, *op. cit.*, pp. 289-293.

VAN RIPER, *op. cit.*, p. 230.

DEEP TESTING

McDONALD, E.: *Articulation Testing and Treatment*. Pittsburgh, Stanwix House, 1964.

VAN RIPER, *op. cit.*, pp. 232-233.

ANALYSIS OF ARTICULATION

VAN RIPER, *op. cit.*, pp. 221-228.

WEST, ANSBERRY, AND CARR, *op. cit.*, pp. 671-678.

Evaluation of Voice

GENERAL EVALUATION

FAIRBANKS, *op. cit.*, p. x.

IRWIN, *op. cit.*, p. 81.

VAN DUSEN, C.: *Training the Voice for Speech*. New York, McGraw, 1953, p. 26.

EVALUATION OF PITCH

ANDERSON (1961), *op. cit.*, pp. 165-166.

FAIRBANKS, *op. cit.*, pp. 122-128.

Johnson, W., Brown, S., Curtis, J., Edney, C., and Keaster, J.:
Speech Handicapped School Children. New York, Harper, 1956,
pp. 554-555.

Van Riper, *op. cit.,* pp. 467-469.

EVALUATION OF RATE

Fairbanks, *op. cit.,* pp. 113-115.

Johnson, Darley, and Spriestersbach, *op. cit.,* pp. 203-236.

EVALUATION OF INTENSITY

Van Riper, *op. cit.,* pp. 469-470.

EVALUATION OF QUALITY

Fairbanks, *op. cit.,* pp. 172-182.

Johnson, Darley, and Spriestersbach, *op. cit.,* pp. 150-158.

Sherman, D.: The merits of backward playing of connected speech
in the scaling of voice quality disorders. *J Speech Hearing Dis,*
*19:*213-321.

Van Riper, *op. cit.,* pp. 470-471.

Evaluation of Stuttering

INITIAL EVALUATION

Johnson, Brown, Curtis, Edney, and Keaster, *op. cit.,* pp. 267-271.

Milisen in Travis, *op. cit.,* p. 298.

Van Riper, *op. cit.,* pp. 485-490.

ASPECTS OF SEVERITY

Johnson, Darley, and Spriestersbach, *op. cit.,* p. 70, pp. 209-217,
pp. 234-235, pp. 281-282 and pp. 291-292.

SPEAKING-TIME LOG

Johnson, Darley, and Spriestersach, *op. cit.,* pp. 214-219.

ATTITUDE AND ADJUSTMENT

Bryngelson, B., Chapman, M., and Hansen, J.: *Know Yourslf.*
Minneapolis, Burgess, 1951, pp. 6-9.

Johnson, Darley, and Spriestersbach, *op. cit.,* pp. 283-290.

Evaluation of Language

GENERAL EVALUATION

Barry, *op. cit.,* pp. 7-8.

Van Riper, *op. cit.,* pp. 127-129.

DIAGNOSTIC EVALUATION

McCarthy, J., and Kirk, S.: *Illinois Test of Psycholinguistic
Abilities.* Urbana, U of Ill, 1961.

Schiefelbush, R. ,and Associates: Language studies of mentally retarded children. *J Speech Hearing Dis* (Monogr), *10,* 1963.

VOCABULARY TEST

AMMONS, R., AND AMMONS, H.: *Full Range Picture Vocabulary Test.* Missoula, Psychological Test Specialists, 1948.

DUNN, L.: *Peabody Picture Vocabulary Test.* 720 Washington Avenue, S.E., Minneapolis, Minnesota, American Guidance.

LANGUAGE DEVELOPMENT MEASURES

CRABTREE, M.: *The Houston Test for Language Development.* P. O. Box 35125, Houston, The Houston Test Company.

JOHNSON, DARLEY, AND SPRIESTERSBACH, *op. cit.,* pp. 167-197.

MECHAM, M.: *Verbal Language Development Scale.* Springfield, Educational Test Bureau, 1959.

TEST FOR APHASIA

EISENSON, HALSTEAD-WEPMAN: *Aphasia Screening Test.* Chicago, Department of Medicine, University of Chicago.

SCHUELL, H.: *Minnesota Test for Differential Diagnosis of Aphasia.* (Research Edition.) Minneapolis, University of Minnesota, Printing Department, 1955.

—————: A short examination for aphasia. *Neurology, VII,* 1957.

WEPMAN, J.: Scale for rating ability in self-correction and recovery from aphasia. *J Speech Hearing Dis, 23,* 1958.

4. Write brief descriptions of the various ways that sibilant sounds may be distorted and list the labels given to these differences by several authorities in speech pathology.

5. Read the medical, psychological and educational reports that are available concerning the clients you have been assigned for this semester. Consult dictionaries of these fields for definitions of the terms you do not understand.

6. Study the physical, psychological and environmental factors that may be related to the speech and language problems of one of your clients by reading from references similar to these:

ADLER, S.: *The Non-Verbal Child.* Springfield, Thomas, 1964.

BARBARA, D.: *Psychological and Psychiatric Aspects of Speech and Hearing.* Springfield, Thomas, 1960.

BOIES, L.: *Fundamentals of Otolaryngology.* Philadelphia, Saunders, 1954.

BLOOM, B.: *Stability and Change in Human Characteristics.* New York, Wiley, 1964.

CRUICKSHANK, W., AND RAUS, G.: *Cerebral Palsy.* Syracuse, Syracuse, 1955.

ERICKSON, E.: *Childhood and Society*. New York, Norton, 1950.

GESSELL, A., AND AMATRUDA, C.: *Developmental Diagnosis*. New York, Hoeber, 1951.

JACKSON C., AND JACKSON, C.: *Diseases of the Nose, Throat, and Ear*. Philadelphia, Saunders, 1945.

JENKINS, G., SHACTER, H., AND BAUER, W.: *These Are Your Children*. Chicago, Scott, 1949.

KANNER, L.: *Child Psychiatry*. Springfield, Thomas, 1948.

LEVIN, N.: *Voice and Speech Disorders: Medical Aspects*. Springfield, Thomas, 1962.

MCCARTHY, D.: Language development in children in Carmichael, L.: *Manual of Child Psychology*. New York, Wiley, 1954.

PENFIELD, W., AND ROBERTS, L.: *Speech and Brain Mechanisms*. Princeton, Princeton U P, 1959.

SARASON, S.: *Psychological Problems in Mental Deficiency*. New York, Harper, 1949.

SCHUELL, H., JENKINS, J., AND JIMENEZ-PABON, E.: *Aphasia in Adults*. New York, Harper, 1964.

SHEEHAN, J.: Conflict theory in stuttering in Eisenson, J.: *Stuttering, A Symposium*. New York, Harper, 1958.

7. Administer some of the following evaluations in order to determine factors that may be related to the speech and language defect of one of your clients:

General Evaluation

CASE HISTORY

BARRY, *op. cit.*, pp. 4-5.

BERRY, M., AND EISENSON, J.: *Speech Disorders*. New York, Appleton, 1956, pp. 525-555.

IRWIN, *op. cit.*, pp. 202-203.

JOHNSON, DARLEY, AND SPRIESTERSBACH, *op. cit.*, pp. 23-69 and pp. 137-149.

MILISEN IN TRAVIS, *op. cit.*, pp. 303-307 and other parts of the chapter.

VAN RIPER, *op. cit.*, pp. 491-502.

OBSERVATION OF BEHAVIOR

GINOTT, H.: *Group Psychotherapy with Children*. New York, McGraw, 1961, pp. 37-50.

HARTLEY, R., FRANK, L., AND GOLDENSON, R.: *Understanding Children's Play*. New York, Columbia, 1952.

MILISEN IN TRAVIS, *op. cit.*, pp. 270-273.

Evaluation of Auditory Factors

SOUND AWARENESS
BARRY, *op. cit.*, p. 6.
AUDITORY MEMORY SPAN
Ibid., p. 7.
BERRY AND EISENSON, *op. cit.*, pp. 503-507.
VAN RIPER, *op. cit.*, p. 477.
WEST, ANSBERRY, AND CARR, *op. cit.*, pp. 657-658.
TEST OF VOCAL PHONICS
VAN RIPER, *op. cit.*, pp. 195-196.
DISCRIMINATION
ANDERSON (1953), *op. cit.*, pp. 323-325.
BARRY, *op. cit.*, pp. 6-7.
BERRY AND EISENSON, *op. cit.*, p. 501.
IRWIN, *op. cit.*, p. 206.
JOHNSON, DARLEY, AND SPRITESTERSBACH, *op. cit.*, pp. 96-98.
PRONOVOST, W., AND DUMBLETON, C.: A picture-type speech sound discrimiation test. *J. Speech Hearing Dis, 18*:258-266.
Seashore Measures of Musical Talent. 304 West 45th Street, New York, The Psychological Corporation.
ANDERSON (1961), *op. cit.*, pp. 436-437.
VAN RIPER, *op. cit.*, p. 478.
WEPMAN, J.: *Auditory Discrimination Test.* 95 East 59th Street, Chicago, Illinois, 1958.

Evaluation of Physical Factors

MOTOR ABILITY
AYERS, A.: *Southern California Motor Accuracy Test.* Box 775, Beverly Hills, California, Western Psychological Services.
BARRY, *op. cit.*, pp. 9-12.
BERRY AND EISENSON, *op. cit.*, pp. 492-493 and pp. 506-508.
IRWIN, *op. cit.*, p. 86.
SPEECH MECHANISM EVALUATION
ANDERSON: *Pinched Throat Test.* 1961, p. 64.
BARRY, *op. cit.*, p. 12.
JOHNSON, DARLEY, AND SPRIESTERSBACH, *op. cit.*, pp. 111-130.
VAN RIPER, *op. cit.*, pp. 472-477 and pp. 481-482.

Evaluation of Mental Factors

FLANAGAN, J.: *SRA Tests of General Ability.* 57 West Grand Avenue,

Chicago, Illinois, Science Research Associates.

GOODENOUGH, F.: *Measurement of Intelligence by Drawings.* Yonkers-on-Hudson, New York, World Book Company.

HISKEY, M.: *Nebraska Test of Learning Aptitude for Young Deaf Children.* New York, Psychological Corporation, 1941.

McMURRY, R.: *SRA Non-verbal Form.* Science Research Associates.

SULLIVAN, E., CLARK, W., AND TIEGS, E.: *California Short-form Test of Mental Maturity* and *California Test of Mental Maturity.* 916 Williamson Street, Madison, Wisconsin, California Test Bureau.

THURSTONE, L., AND THURSTONE, T.: *SRA Primary Mental Abilities Test.* Science Research Associates.

Evaluation of Social, Emotional and Environmental Factors

DERI, S.: *Szondi Test.* (Personality picture test.) New York, Grune, 1949.

DOLL, E.: *Vineland Social Maturity Scale.* Minneapolis, Educational Test Bureau, 1947.

REMMERS, H., AND SHINBERG, B.: *SRA Youth Inventory.* Science Research Associates, 1950.

ROGERS, C.: *Personality Adjustment Inventory.* 291 Broadway, New York, Association Press.

TRAVIS-JOHNSTON: *Projection Test.* 544 West Colorado Boulevard, Glendale, California, Griffin-Patterson Company.

THORPE, L., CLARK, W., AND TIEGS, E.: *California Test of Personality.* Calfiornia Test Bureau.

WILEY, J.: A scale to measure parental attitudes. *J Speech Hearing Dis, 20,* 1955.

8. Summarize the information that you obtained from evaluating the speech and language abilities of a client and the factors that may be related to these abilities by using forms similar to those listed in these references:

CYPREANSEN, WILEY, AND LAASE, *op. cit.,* pp. 325-334.

IRWIN, *op. cit.,* p. 93.

JOHNSON, DARLEY, AND SPRIESTERSBACH, *op. cit.,* pp. 333-337.

VAN RIPER, *op. cit.,* p. 234.

9. Construct a form to use when observing and evaluating diagnostic sessions. Use the form when observing at least five such sessions.

10. Construct a chart (or write a paper) which will assist

you in making the differential diagnosis which you find the most difficult.

11. Arrange to view some of the following films:

Titles: *The Auditorially Handicapped Child*
      Speech Disorders: Physical Handicaps
Distributor: Audio-Visual Center
      Indiana University
      Bloomington, Indiana

Titles: *Examining the Oral Mechanism*
      New Hope for Stutterers
      A Survey of Children's Speech Disorders
Distributor: Bureau of Audio-Visual Instruction
      State University of Iowa
      Iowa City, Iowa

Titles: *Basic Audiometric Testing*
      Introductory Examination of the Aphasic
Distributor: Bureau of Audio-Visual Instruction
      University of Wisconsin
      1312 West Johnson Street
      Madison 6, Wisconsin

Titles: *Speech Evaluation of an Adult Post-Operative*
      Cleft Palate Patient
Distributor: M. D. Foundation
      6252 Primrose Avenue
      Hollywood 28, California

Title: *A Psycho-Educational Evaluation of Severely*
      Involved Children
Distributor: United Cerebral Palsy Association
      321 West 44th Street
      New York, New York

Title: *Clinical Examination Procedure*
Distributor: Audio-Visual Center
      Syracuse University
      Syracuse, New York

12. Discuss with your colleagues the following report of a language evaluation. If the samples obtained were representative of Mary's abilities, what, in your opinion, is her present language age? What additional interviewing, testing, counseling, etc., needs to be attempted? Or what recommendations would you make?

A relatively unstructured evaluation of some aspects of Mary Jones' general behavior and language abilities was attempted. She was four years old at the time of the evaluation.

Mrs. Jones was present, because Mary seemed reluctant to enter the testing room without her mother; however, Mary seldom noticed her mother during the evaluation period. She enjoyed playing with a toy man made of rubber whose ears, mouth and nose protruded and who squeaked when she squeezed him. The examiner gave her this toy when her attention wandered from the tasks being presented. Mary imitated some of the examiner's actions and words; for example, she removed dominoes from a toy truck and repeated the word "more" each time the examiner said, "more dominoes." She did not imitate the actions of stacking the dominoes or of placing them end-to-end even when verbal instructions were given. After playing with the dominoes she sat in a chair when the examiner patted the seat of the chair and she scribbled on a sheet of paper with a crayon. She pretended to talk into a toy telephone, holding it in proper position, but did not vocalize in answer to questions such as, "How are you, Mary?" She placed blocks on a stand after being helped and took the blocks off and put them on several times without assistance while repeating the words "on" and "off" after the examiner. When Mary's back was toward the examiner she placed her hand on her back. Mary did not want the examiner to touch her, but did not react to her hand as she would have to an object.

Parts of the following subtests of the Illinois Test of Psycholinguistic Abilities were presented. Mary made no responses that could be scored.

Subtest	
Visual Decoding (demonstration item only)	Attempted to tear the picture from the book.
Motor Encoding	Hammered the dominoes using her left hand. (Repeated the action many times.) Drank from the toy pitcher and cup. Handled the toy gun. Did not imitate the examiner pouring from pitcher to cup.
Visual Motor Sequencing	Attempted to tear the picture chips apart. Later used them as saucers for the toy cup and pitcher.
Auditory Vocal Sequencing	Did not repeat the two digits said by the examiner.

Some items from the Parsons Language Sample were presented. The results were:

Tact	No verbal response to the objects.
Echoic	Said "ball" after examiner said, "Say ball." Said "boy" after examiner said, "Say cowboy." No other responses.
Echoic Gesture	Pointed to the light after examiner had pointed and said, "Do this." Rubbed the top of her head perhaps a minute or more after examiner had performed the same action and said, "Do this."
Comprehension	Turned to face the examiner after examiner said her name. Gave the examiner a toy when examiner held her hand out with the palm up. Placed her fingers on the cup when examiner gave the direction.
Intraverbal	No response given to the first question—which was the only one asked.
Intraverbal Gestural	Repeated the word "light" when asked "where is the light?"

Mary cooperated fairly well during the evaluation which lasted approximately an hour. At one time she pushed several toys off the table.

Comments made by the mother: Mary does not like anyone to touch her. She does not sleep well. She rocks back and forth on her bed before going to sleep. It often takes her quite awhile to get to sleep. Mother is afraid younger sister will imitate Mary's speech. Mary said her first words at nine months and carried out verbal directions at one year. Her speech did not seem to improve after she was two years old. Some time ago, Mary would hit her head against her crib when she did not get her way. This behavior has since changed to pushing over chairs or ripping paper and throwing things.

Chapter III

CREATING AN ATMOSPHERE

T HERAPISTS WHO ARE understanding, helpful and self-confident frequently create an atmosphere in which clients improve their speech and language and often their personalities. Some authorities believe that the interaction between the therapist and the client is the most important element in therapy. They believe that taking an interest in and becoming involved with a client is more important than the procedures or methods that are used.

SKILLFUL THERAPISTS ARE UNDERSTANDING

Skillful therapists understand their clients and often develop

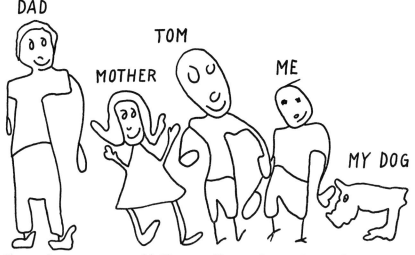

Drawn by a seven-year-old "functional" articulation client when he was asked to draw a picture of "the people who live at your house."

a client-centered relationship with them. They may develop the relationship by following the teachings of Carl Rogers. (See Suggestion One at the close of the chapter.) They accept the client as he is, are interested in him, respect him, attempt to see things as he sees them and regard him positively. They frequently communicate understanding of the client's feelings by restating his remarks and by attempting to express his unexpressed feelings. If they are not specifically trained in client-centered therapy, and realize that they are spending most of the therapy time talking with the client about his feelings, they refer him to a trained counselor and, if it seems advisable, discontinue speech therapy temporarily. Experienced therapists are often skilled in accepting a client's behavior and feelings even when they are not acquainted with his case history. They realize that his behavior and feelings reflect the present and past conditions of his organism, his personality and his environment.

Many beginning therapists become more accepting after they have increased their knowledge of the client and his problem. They increase their knowledge of the client by becoming familiar with his case history, trying to understand his feelings and the individual aspects of his problem. (See Chapter I, sections on Knowledge of the Problem and Knowledge of the Client.)

A client-centered relationship may be developed when indirect as well as when direct speech therapy is used. A therapist who was using indirect speech therapy with fourteen perschool children tried to reflect their feelings at the close of the therapy period when they were waiting for their mothers to come for them.

Therapist: You like to get close to the door when the movie is finished because you know your mother will be here soon. You want to be the first one to leave, Johnny. You wonder why your mother hasn't come and you wish she would hurry. You've been here a long time. You want to get home to eat lunch and to play.

After the children realized that the therapist understood some of their feelings, they seemed more willing to sit on their chairs while waiting for their mothers. This therapist had some difficulty establishing a helping relationship with George, who was cerebral palsied. She realized that she didn't like George very much and she tried to discover the basis of the difficulty. She decided that George frequently got in her way. He wanted his shoe tied or his name tag pinned on or he tried to find other children's name tags. She decided to give George an interesting puzzle or toy to play with when she was distributing name tags. She also tried to express the interest she did have in him and tried to empathize with him. After a few weeks had elapsed, his mother stated that she didn't know what had happened to George, but he was enjoying therapy more and was eager to come each day.

Another therapist attempted to use some client-centered therapy techniques with a client who was having direct therapy. A university-aged client with a German dialect who planned to return to Germany to teach English had been working for a number of sessions to improve her production of [θ] and [ð]. She could produce these sounds acceptably in conversational speech, but according to her own statements and statements of her friends she was not using the sounds outside of therapy. The following is a report of one of the sessions the therapist held to determine whether or not the client's feelings were interfering with carry-over.

Therapist: How do you think you're getting along in therapy?
Hedwig: Oh, very well, I think.
Therapist: You believe your progress is satisfactory.
Hedwig: Yes, I can make the sounds we've been working on. I can produce them in words and sentences but I seldom use them when I'm not at the clinic.
Therapist: You can produce the "th" sounds, but you seldom use them outside the clinic.
Hedwig: That's right. I don't like to use them when I talk with my friends.
Therapist: You'd rather not produce these sounds the "new way" when you talk with people.
Hedwig: It feels strange and besides I don't like to make these sounds the way you and other American speakers make

them. I feel as though I'm sticking my tongue out at the people I'm talking to and I've been taught that this is rude.

The therapist believed that Hedwig would not have progressed if she had kept this attitude toward the acceptable production of these sounds. The therapist could have tried to have talked her out of her attitude, but instead she understood and accepted her feelings, reexpressed them for her and let Hedwig talk herself out of her feelings. Hedwig finally decided that she could look in the mirror and modfiy her production of the "th" sounds, that she would notice how her American friends produced the sounds, and that perhaps she wasn't using as much tongue protrusion as she had thought. After her attitude changed, her progress in carry-over was satisfactory.

Another therapist was working directly with a group of university-aged stutterers. One member of the group, Bob, had been required to attend speech therapy in the public schools for more than ten years. They were using the mirror to analyze the visual aspects of their stuttering. Bob had not participated in the session and the therapist failed to sense the feelings that were beginning to build up in him. He started laughing at the others in the group. The therapist ignored his laughter and proceeded with the session. Finally he said, "Can't you see your toe nails? They curl when you have a block. Why do we sit here looking at ourselves? I'm not going to do any more of this." He became very angry, paced the floor, shouted that he had never had a therapist who knew anything about stutterers or who understood how they felt and that he didn't believe in the theory we were advocating. He ran out of the room shouting that he would never return. The therapist decided to ignore his actions for a few weeks. When he did not return to therapy, she sent him the following letter:

Dear Bob,

Sometimes we do things and say things in therapy that you do not agree with. You think that mirror work is a waste of time and that our ideas are false. It isn't necessary for you to believe the way we do in order to come to therapy sessions. Next week we shall discuss Sheehan's theory of stuttering and analyze some of the problems of members of the group as they relate to his theory. We will probably continue the discussions for a few weeks. You are welcome to come to any of these sessions, but if you had rather not come you will not be required to attend.

Sincerely,
Betty Jones

He returned to therapy in a few weeks and after a few sessions became an interested participant.

Sometimes beginning therapists have difficulty in establishing satisfactory relationships with clients. One therapist said that it was easier for her to think of an adult aphasic client as a father than as a client and a young college-aged client as a friend rather than a client. After she recognized these tendencies, she was able to establish somewhat more satisfactory relationships with these clients.

SKILLFUL THERAPISTS ARE HELPFUL

Some clients seem to profit more from an indirect approach to speech therapy than from a direct approach. When a therapist uses an indirect approach, the client may be unaware that he has a speech problem. What the client says is more important than how he says it, and the client has fun talking. When a therapist uses a direct approach, the client is first convinced that his speech needs improving and a program involving ear training and drills is used. The objective is often the improvement of the production of sounds, one at a time. Some clients are not ready for a direct approach because they are too immature, or listeners have been too critical of their speech, or they do not have a desire to communicate. A direct approach is usually used when the client wants to communicate, can accept direction and has a normal language structure and mental ability. Therapists should probably have used indirect therapy with two five-year-old delayed speech clients. One little girl had direct speech therapy twice a week in a speech clinic and once a week in her public school. She often chewed her fingers and chewed holes in the collars of her dresses. When the direct therapy was discontinued, she became more relaxed and stopped chewing her fingers and her clothing. The other little girl seemed shy and had not profited from a semester of direct therapy. Her new therapist did not mention her defective sounds, but asked her to bring her doll to therapy. The therapist and the client enjoyed playing and talking together. They had tea parties and played *Come to See.* When the client misarticulated a sound of a word, the therapist articulated the word correctly in a short meaningful sentence. The client's desire and ability to communicate improved. Some five-year-old clients, however, can profit from direct therapy. A therapist used an indirect approach with a five-year-old client until she said, "When are we going to stop playing games and get to work on my speech. You know I can't make some of my sounds right."

An indirect approach is often used in the carry-over stage of therapy. One group of college-aged stutterers had worked directly on their problem for two semesters. They believed that they needed more therapy, but did not wish to continue with the procedures they had been using. They decided to meet once a week to talk about their experiences, give book reviews, exchange ideas about current events and discuss controversial questions.

Therapists create atmospheres that are suited to the approach. The following descriptions illustrate some of the differences between the atmosphere of an indirect therapy session and the atmosphere of a direct therapy session.

An Indirect Therapy Session

Fourteen preschool children with articulation and delayed speech problems are seated in a semicircle in front of the therapist. The therapist asks the children who have pet kittens to tell about them. She then tells a story about an angry kitten (using a kitten puppet).

Therapist: Sometimes the kitten forgets to say [f, f, f] when he is angry and he says [s, s, s]. Put on your listening ears. (Children place their hands behind their ears.) When the angry kitten says [f, f, f] nod your head. When he says [s, s, s] shake your head. (Children follow the directions as therapist continues to tell the story.)

Therapist: Who would like to play like he's the angry kitten?

Debbie: I would. (Debbie puts the kitten puppet on her hand.) She says [f, f, f]. (Other children pretent that they are the angry kitten. No attempt is made to improve the children's production of the [f] sound.)

Therapist: Who wants to help me tell the story of *Jack and the Beanstalk*? (Johnny raises his hand. He places cutouts of the characters from the story on the felt board, as the therapist and he tell a simplified version of the story.)

Therapist: What did the giant say?

Children: Fee, Fi, Fo, Fum, I smell the blood of an Englishman.

Therapist: Bobby, will you pretend that you are the giant. (Bobby repeats the giant's speech. Other children pretend that they are the giant. Therapist finishes the story.)

Therapist: Now, we'll play *Farmer in the Dell*.

A Direct Therapy Session

(Five seven-year-old children with distorted sibilants are each seated in front of a mirror. In previous sessions, they had come to the conclusion that they needed to improve their production of [s].)

Therapist: Make [s] five times. Listen closely because I'm going to have you tell what you sound like when you make this sound. Each child produces [s] five times.) Jack, how do you sound when you make [s]?

Jack: I almost whistle.

Therapist: Is there anything else you'd like to tell us?

Jack: I make it too long. I'd like to say it in a shorter time. (The other children describe how their [s] sounds.)

Therapist: Watch yourself carefully in the mirror as you make [s] five times. Can you see your tongues? Where is your tongue, Betty?

Betty: My tongue is close to my upper teeth. (Each child describes the position of his tongue when he produces [s].)

Therapist: Try changing where you put your tongue and listen to your [s] sound. Keep trying different things until you get a [s] sound that you like better than the sound you made when you came in today. When you want us to listen, tell us and we'll see how we like it.

Sometimes direct therapy sessions are rather dull, especially when emphasis is placed on drill that the client does not understand. The therapist may, however, create an atmosphere that is relaxing and enjoyable and also attain the objectives of the session. The following description of a stuttering therapy session conducted by the late Wendall Johnson with five children, who were approximately nine years old was an enjoyable and profitable session. (Permission granted by Johnson to include the description.)

Another Direct Therapy Session

Johnson: What do you do in therapy that helps you most?

Dorothy: Talk with people.

Johnson: What would you do for the rest of the summer if you were planning the therapy?

Dennis: Use more eye contact.

William: Fake stuttering sometimes.

Bobby: Read to myself because I'm not so bothered then.

George: Talk with strangers.

Johnson: Who are these strangers? Do they live in "Strangeria"? Do they have three eyes? Who are strangers?

George: People I haven't seen before.

Dennis: They could be strangers in one way and not in another.

Johnson: How?

Dennis: Well, I might have seen them before, but I might not know their names.

Johnson: Do any of you *know* any strangers?

(The children laugh.)

Bobby: We should get to know them as soon as possible, I guess.

Johnson: It's a funny thing about strangers—as soon as you get to know them they turn into friends!

(Each child reads orally. George blocks on the word China.)

Johnson: What are you doing?

George: Stuttering.

(Further questions by Johnson as George continues his silent block.)

George: I'm putting my tongue behind my teeth and keeping it there.

Johnson: Keep doing what you're doing until you decide to do something else. You could do something like this.

(Johnson reads and rereads the sentence containing China, using different patterns of repetition and prolongation of the sounds of the word. The last time he reads it he pauses before the word China, walks over to the window, looks out, turns around and then says the word. The children laugh.)

Johnson: Don't call it stuttering. Call it killing time until you say China. You don't have to work at killing time. It's like waiting for the bus—you just stand and wait. Have fun with a book, seeing how many ways you can kill time before you say words.

Therapists often help clients by attempting to influence the behavior of persons who are in contact with the client.

A therapist noticed, during one of the parents' visiting days at a summer residential camp, that the mother of a young client

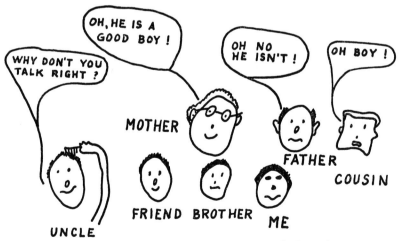

Drawn by a nine-year-old stutterer when he was asked to draw a picture of himself, his family, and friends, and to indicate what they might say about him.

with delayed speech seldom talked with him. Another therapist heard a mother say that she hoped her fourteen-year-old daughter could be fitted with an eye glass hearing aid so that the new friends she met when she entered junior high would not know that she was hard-of-hearing. The therapist realized that a new aid would not conceal the client's many speech differences and the difficulties she had in understanding others. These therapists were angry with the mothers and wanted to tell them that what they were doing was wrong. Fortunately, however, the therapists realized that they should talk the problems over with the supervisor. The supervisor accepted the clinicians' feelings and decided to talk with the mother of the younger child and to write a letter to the school social worker who had been working with the mother of the older client, because she realized that it would take many hours or perhaps years of counseling before this mother would be able to accept her daughter's differences.

Report of the Interview

The supervisor encouraged Mrs. Daniels to talk about Charles and his speech problem. When Mrs. Daniels described her feelings and actions toward Charles, the supervisor did not evaluate them. This seemed to establish rapport, encouraged Mrs. Daniels to talk more freely and to ask what caused Charles' problem. The supervisor said that with most clients there are many factors related to the problem. She named some of the more common causes of delayed speech and asked Mrs. Daniels which ones she believed had influenced the development of Charles' problem. She decided that her being away from home at work had contributed to it. She also stated that she talked very little to him when she was at home because she was tired and it was often hard for her to understand him. The supervisor gave Mrs. Daniels the following suggestions because she seemed anxious to know what she could do and willing to try to help Charles:

1. When you can't understand Charles, ask him to tell you more or show you what he wants;
2. Talk with him about what you are doing, using short but complete sentences;
3. Describe orally some of his actions and apparent feelings.

Some parents, teachers and others have the ability, time and interest to enable them to be quite helpful. Many therapists organize parent groups and conduct training programs for parents and teachers. Sometimes, however, it seems necessary for the client to learn to adjust to the behavior of persons who are in his environment.

SKILLED THERAPISTS ARE SELF-CONFIDENT

Skilled therapists believe that the procedures they are using are helpful, they enjoy their work and they are good disciplinarians. A beginning therapist was afraid that the procedures she was using with a stutterer were ineffective. Some of her feelings were evidently communicated to her client because he asked that a different therapist be assigned to him because, "She doesn't know what she is doing." An artist once stated that observers enjoyed most the paintings that he had thoroughly enjoyed painting. It seems that clients enjoy working with therapists who like their work. Therapists become better disciplinarians when they realize that they need to be kind but firm. The establishment of a client-centered relationship and the use of sound educational practices also help. This part of the chapter will include some examples of practices that were effective for some therapists. One therapist was more stimulating, lively and active when working with quiet or depressed clients, but used a slower rate of speaking and acted more deliberately when working with hyperactive clients. She often arranged for hyperactive groups to have activities that were focused and that kept their hands busy. She discovered, too, that both groups like a variety of pace. Another therapist tried to suit the methods of discipline to the type of approach she was using. When working indirectly with a group of preschoolers, she found that it was difficult to keep the children sitting on their chairs during listening time. One session, she gave each child an imaginary bottle of paste and a brush, and each spread paste on the seat of his chair before sitting down. They enjoyed this pretend activity and they seemed more willing to remain seated.

Would you like to become more understanding, helpful and

self-confident? The following suggestions are presented to help you improve your skill in creating a desirable atmosphere.

Suggestions for Improving Skill in Creating an Atmosphere

1. Take the Pre-test in Poter, E.: *An Introduction to Therapeutic Counseling.* Boston, Houghton, 1950, for an indication of your ability as a counselor. Read from references similar to the following and then take the Post-test in Poter to see if your ability has improved:

AXLINE, V.: *Play Therapy.* Boston, Houghton, 1947.

DESPERT, J.: *Play analysis.* In Nolan, N., and Pacella, B. (eds.): *Modern Trends in Child Psychiatry.* New York, Int. Univs., 1945.

EVRAIFF, W.: *Helping Counselors Grow Professionally.* Englewood Cliffs, Prentice-Hall.

GINOTT, H.: *Group Psychotherapy with Children.* New York, McGraw, 1961.

HOBBS, N.: Client-centered psychotherapy. In McCarey, J. (ed.): *Six Approaches to Psychotherapy.* New York, Dryden Press, 1955.

LIPPMAN, H.: *Treatment of the Child in Emotional Conflict.* New York, McGraw, 1956.

MOUSTAKAS, C.: *Children in Play Therapy.* New York, McGraw, 1953.

ROGERS, C.: *Client-Centered Therapy.* Boston, Houghton, 1950.

—————: *On Becoming a Person.* Cambridge, The Riverside Press, 1961.

SLAVSON, S.: *Child Psychotherapy.* New York, Columbia, 1952.

—————: Group psychotherapies. In McCarey, J. (ed.): *Six Approaches to Psychotherapy.* New York, Dryden Press, 1955.

SNYDER, W.: *Casebook of Non-Directive Counseling.* Boston, Houghton, 1947.

—————: *The Psychotherapy Relationship.* New York, Macmillan, 1961.

2. Read from references similar to the following to help you improve your ability to apply some of the principles of client-centered therapy to Speech Therapy:

BACKUS, O.: Group structure in speech therapy. In Travis, L. (ed.): *Handbook of Speech Pathology.* New York, Appleton, 1957.

HEJNA, R.: *Interviews with a Stutterer.* Box 1713, Ann Arbor, Michigan, Speech Materials.

—————: *Speech Disorders and Nondirective Therapy.* New York, Ronald, 1960.

MARTIN, E.: Client-centered therapy as a theoretical orientation for speech therapy. *ASHA,* April, 1963, 576-578.

MURPHY, A., AND FITZSIMONS, R.: *Stuttering and Personality Dynamics.* New York, Ronald, 1960.

THORNE, D.: Client-centered therapy for voice and personality cases, *J Speech Hearing Dis, 12*:314-318.

3. Listen to the recording of passages from the counseling experience of a stutterer. *The Case of Jim.* Distributor: Counselor Recordings, Box 6184, Acklen Station, Nashville 12, Tennessee.

4. Deepen your understanding of your clients and/or yourself by studying references similar to these:

ALMY, M.: *Ways of Studying Children, A Manual for Teachers.* New York, Columbia, 1959.

ALSCHULER, R., AND HATTWICK, L.: *Painting and Personality.* Chicago, U of Chicago, 1947.

BOWER, E.: *Early Identification of Emotionally Handicapped Children in School.* Springfield, Thomas, 1960.

BRYNGELSON, B.: *Personality Development Through Speech.* Minneapolis, Denison, 1964.

CARLSON, E.: *Born That Way.* New York, Day, 1941. (Autobiography of a cerebral palsied individual.)

KRAKOWSKI, A., AND SANTORA, D. (eds.): *Child Psychiatry and the General Practitioner. Diagnosis and Treatment of Emotional Diseases of Childhood.* Springfield, Thomas, 1962.

MALAMUD, D., AND MACHOVER, S.: *Toward Self-Understanding.* Springfield, Thomas, 1964.

MENNINGER, W.: *Growing Up Emotionally.* Chicago, Science Research Associates, 1957. (A booklet.)

————: Self-understanding, a first step to understanding children. Chicago, Science Research Associates, 1951. (A booklet.)

WARFIELD, F.: *Cotton In My Ears.* New York, Viking, 1942. (Autobiography of a hard-of-hearing individual.)

WHITE, V.: *Studying the Individual Pupil.* New York, Harper, 1958.

5. Read Hahn, E.: Indications for direct, nondirect, and indirect methods in speech correction. *J Speech Hearing Dis, 26*:230-236, 1961, before deciding which approach to use with each of your clients this semester.

6. Plan and conduct an interview with the parents of one of

your clients after you consult references similar to these:

ELLIS, A.: *How to Live With a Neurotic*. New York, Crown.

EWING, I., AND EWING, A.: *New Opportunities for Deaf Children*. Springfield, Thomas, 1964.

GLIDEWELL, J.: *Parental Attitudes and Child Behavior*. Springfield, Thomas, 1961.

IRWIN, R.: *A Speech Pathologist Talks to Parents and Teachers*. Pittsburgh, Stanwix House.

McDONALD, E.: *Understanding Those Feelings*. Pittsburgh, Stanwix House.

MENNINGER, W., and others: *How to Help Your Children; the Parents Handbook*. New York, Sterling, 1959.

SMITH, B.: *No Language But a Cry*. Boston, Beacon Press. (Concerns the emotionally disturbed.)

WYATT, G.: Treating children with nonorganic language disorders and Treatment of stuttering children and their parents. Wellesley Hills, Massachusetts, Wellesley Public Schools.

7. Write a short, clear and informative statement for distribution to classroom teachers on a topic such as: Children with non-fluent speech; Helping the hard of hearing child in the classroom.

8. Collect material similar to that listed below and distribute it to parents and/or teachers who, in your opinion, can use it effectively:

ALLODI, F., LEE, L., AND LIEBMAN, E.: *Building Blocks for Speech*. 225 Greenwood Boulevard, Evanston, Illinois, Junior League. (For use with very young children.)

BARUCH, D.: *New Ways in Discipline*. New York, McGraw, 1947.

BATTIN, R., AND HAUG, C.: *Speech and Language Delay*: *A Home Training Program*. Springfield, Thomas, 1964.

BOLAND, L., AND JONES, M.: *Mike and Cindy Stories*. Edmond, Central College Press, 1965.

BYRNE, M.: *The Child Speaks*: *A Speech Improvement Program for Kindergarten and First Grade*. New York, Harper.

CUTTS, N., AND MOSELEY, N.: *Teaching the Disorderly Pupil in Elementary and Secondary School*. 750 Third Avenue, New York, David McKay Company.

JONES, M.: *Speech Correction at Home*. Springfield, Thomas, 1957.

PALMER, C.: *Speech and Hearing Problems*: *A Guide for Parents and Teachers*. Springfield, Thomas, 1961.

SINGER, P.: *Speak Up.* 501 Main Street West, Rochester, New York, Hearing and Speech Center.

WARKOMSKI AND IRWIN: *Play and Say.* Pittsburgh, Stanwix House.

Pamphlets from sources such as these:

National Association for Mental Health
10 Columbus Circle
New York 19, New York
Rehabilitation Literature
2023 West Ogden Avenue
Chicago 12, Illinois
Ross Laboratories
Columbus 16, Ohio
Science Research Associates
259 East Erie Street
Chicago 11, Illinois
The Volta Bureau
1537 35th Street N.W.
Washington, D. C.

9. Make a collection of lists of audio-visual materials that may be used with parents and teachers of clients. Obtain them from sources such as these:

American Speech and Hearing Association
9030 Old Georgetown Rd.
Washington, D. C.
Beltone Company
47th Street near Vanderbuilt Plaza
New York, New York
Council for Exceptional Children
1201 16th Street N.W.
Washington, D. C.
John Tracy Clinic
806 West Adams Boulevard
Los Angeles 7, California
National Society for Crippled Children and Adults
2023 W. Ogden Avenue
Chicago, Illinois
Veterans Administration, Central Office
Washington, D. C.

10. The following descriptions were given orally by five high school aged stutterers after they listened to tape recordings

of their conversational speech. Write out statements which will reflect their feelings:

Description I

When I stutter I feel very tense throughout my body, especially in my chest. My chest just tightens up and also I feel tense in my legs. The problem I have the most is with certain sounds which I can't pronounce. I also have a lot of trouble in starting a sentence. The first word is what I usually block on the most. The word comes out in sections. First I have a block on the first part of the word and then on the second part of the word. I get very nervous when I talk and sometimes the words don't come out at all.

Description II

When I do not substitute words I have more stuttering and longer blocks. I can speak fluently if I reduce my rate of speaking and try to relax, but I'm not satisfied with this deliberate speech pattern. It may be okay for a public speech but not for everyday speech—that which is most essential in everyday life.

Description III

My voice sounds worse to me than it has for a long time. I noticed I have trouble breathing as well as talking. Sometimes I breathe in when saying a word. Other times I try to take a deep breath first, but after I say one or two words I am short of breath. My voice sounds very rough to me. I can't seem to talk smoothly and my throat feels tense. I noticed that when I stopped and tried to relax it still sounded tense.

Description IV

After listening to my talking I must say that I would hate to have people listen to me when I sound this way. I seem all choked up. My voice was shaky. My blocks come mostly at the beginning of sentences. I do not particularly like the sound of my voice. It reminds me of someone who I do not like.

Description V

I talk better here in the clinic than I do outside because

there is no feeling of hostility or being overcriticized as there often is other places, expecially in a strange situation. Because it does not bother me as much, I do not think I stutter as much. I think that during a block the worst part is not the sound but the distorted facial expression which doesn't show on tape. I have found I can eliminate many blocks by talking rapidly. This sounds almost as bad as a block. Through listening to myself I have found out how I sound to others and that even in a severe block I can make myself understood.

11. Plan a series of conferences with the parents of a child who is beginning to stutter. Read references similar to the following before developing your plan:

SHAMES, G., AND SHERRICK, C.: A discussion of non-fluency and stuttering as operant behavior. *J Speech Hearing Dis, 28*:3-18, 1963.

12. After reading the following report of part of an interview with a parent, decide what further questions should be asked and/or what recommendations should be made.

ANN WALLACE, *Interviewer and Reporter*
October 10, 1963

Re: Interview with John Jamison's mother.

Purpose: To obtain more information about John and his behavior.

Mrs. Jamison stated that a professor in the Education Department had given John an IQ test and had told her that John was retarded about one year.

John has three older sisters and a younger brother. His relationship with them is satisfactory according to Mrs. Jamison; however, she said he is sometimes in conflict with Joan, his youngest sister, who is now ten years old. He scratches and shakes her. When asked how often this occurs she said, "Well, not **every** evening." He apparently dislikes his younger brother, Tommy, who is two years old. According to Mrs. Jamison, her husband is partial to Tommy and John resents this. He often shows his resentment by biting Tommy. His contacts with children his age is limited because they live on a farm, and they have been further limited by his mother. Children laugh at him or ignore him or he annoys them and for these reasons she does not encourage his playing with other children. He does attend Sunday School and seems to enjoy it and likes his present teacher very much.

He has difficulty expressing his thoughts and feelings. (He does not use sentences.) He has communicated more recently since he has had a new pet dog.

Interviewer administered part of the Vineland Social Maturity Scale and found that John's social age is between four and five years. He is chronologically five years two months old.

Chapter IV

USING PROCEDURES

Skilled therapists utilize procedures that are related to the client's problem, focused and challenging. After a therapist decides whether she will use a direct or an indirect approach, she determines what steps she and the client may take to improve his speech and language, which of these should be taken and how difficult they should be.

PROCEDURES RELATED TO THE PROBLEM

The client's problem may be divided into the aspects that

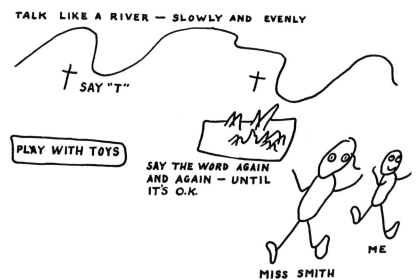

Drawn in answer to the question, "What do we do in speech class?" by a nine-year-old client with ataxia.

are related to speech problems in general and the aspects that are related to a particular type of speech defect. Therapists formulate objectives and use procedures related to these aspects of the problem.

Therapists formulate objectives and use procedures related to speech problems in general. They may be similar to these:

Objectives	*Procedures*
1. To obtain information about the client.	1. Administer additional diagnostic evaluations. (See Chapter II, "Using Diagnostic Tools.")
2. To create a helping relationship.	2. Restate the client's feelings, etc. (See Chapter III, "Creating an Atmosphere.")
3. To motivate the client.	3. Participate in enjoyable activities involving speech. Play tape recordings of the client's speech. Keep speaking-time records.
4. To minimize the influence of causal factors.	4. Refer client to appropriate professional personnel. Confer with persons who are in contact with the client. (See Chapter III, "Creating an Atmosphere.")

Therapists formulate objectives and use procedures related to the particular type of speech defect the client possesses.

If the client has an articulation defect, the therapist may formulate objectives and use procedures similar to these:

Objectives	*Procedures*
1. To improve ability to hear sounds.	1. Isolate, identify and discriminate sounds.
2. To improve functioning of the articulators.	2. Exercise articulators.
3. To use acceptable sound production habitually.	3. Produce acceptable sounds in simple contexts. Strengthen acceptable sound production.

If the client has a voice defect, the therapist may formulate objectives and use procedures similar to these:

Objectives	*Procedures*
1. To relax the body and the vocal mechanism.	1. Take relaxation exercises.
2. To improve auditory discrimination between types of vocal characteristics.	2. Administer auditory training.
3. To improve functioning of the articulators.	3. Exercise articulators.
4. To determine characteristics of the new voice.	4. Vary vocal production and evaluate the results.
5. To use new voice in conversational speech.	5. Produce new voice in simple contexts. Produce new voice in complex contexts. Produce new voice in easy and difficult situations.

If an older client stutters, the therapist may formulate objectives and use procedures similar to these:

Objectives	*Procedures*
1. To improve attitude toward stuttering.	1. Discuss attitude toward stuttering. Define and give examples of an objective attitude.
2. To improve self-concept and attitude toward others.	2. Discuss client's personality. Observe listener's reactions to stuttering. Interview listeners.
3. To increase understanding of stuttering.	3. Present information about stuttering. Read books and/or articles on stuttering.
4. To develop communication skills that are not related to stuttering.	4. Increase amount of time spent in speaking. Use more eye contact.
5. To decrease stuttering symptoms.	5. Compare normal speakers' disfluencies with stuttering blocks. Describe the visual and auditory aspects of the client's stuttering. Modify the visual and auditory aspects of the client's stuttering.

If the client has a language problem, the therapist may formulate objectives and use procedures similar to these:

Objectives	*Procedures*
1. To increase awareness of environment and ability to organize experiences.	1. Recognize differences and similarities in form, color, size, function, etc., of objects.
2. To increase awareness of self.	2. Recognize and identify parts of the body.
3. To improve receptive language.	3. Recognize the names of objects, persons and actions. Follow oral directions. Listen to stories.
4. To improve expressive language.	4. Identify objects, persons and actions by names. Use verbs, pronouns, prepositions, etc., more acceptably. Use complete sentences to express thoughts and feelings. Verbalize abstractions.

PROCEDURES THAT ARE FOCUSED

The objectives and procedures presented in the preceeding section of the chapter are stated in general terms. When working with a particular client, the therapist uses concrete objectives and procedures and limits the number according to the abilities of the client and the time available.

When helping clients with articulation defects, beginning therapists sometimes have difficulty deciding which sound or sounds to improve first. Some of them spend a semester correcting a [t/θ] or a [d/ð] substitution, even though the client lives in a dialect region where these substitutions are common. It seems doubtful that much time should ever be spent on them as the intelligibility of the client's speech is probably only slightly affected by these substitutions.

Therapists often answer questions such as these in order to determine which sound to improve first:

Which defective sound will be easiest to correct? Which sound is acceptably produced inconsistently or following stimulation? Which sound is the easiest for clients in general to produce? Which one is produced first in normal speech development? Which one does the client wish to correct? Which one has been criticized by listeners? And which one will improve intelligibility most?

A therapist was working with five 9-year-old boys who had functional articulation defects and had had two years of speech therapy. They could not produce the [l] and [r] in some words and the incorrect production of these sounds seemed to be contributing to the indistinctness of their speech. The therapist listed the following objectives and samples of the procedures she intended to use:

Objectives	*Procedures*
1. To improve ability to discriminate between [w] and [l] and [w] and [r].	1. Play a space game using the auditory training unit. (Discrimination exercises.)
2. To produce [l] and [r] in words and nonsense syllables.	2. Play space game using key words containing [l] and [r]. Play checkers using nonsense syllables formed from parts of the key words, other nonsense syllables and other words containing [l] and [r].
3. To produce [l] and [r] habitually.	3. Tape record mock broadcasts of baseball games. Write and read original science fiction stories.

A therapist decided to use therapy based on Van Riper's theory of stuttering with four university-aged stutterers who had had therapy in high school. Their high school therapy was based on theories other than Van Riper's. The following objectives and procedures were used with them:

Objectives	*Procedures*
1. To create a helping relationship.	1. Converse about interests. Discuss attitudes toward stuttering.
2. To obtain information about the clients stuttering.	2. Measure frequency, adaptation and consistency of stuttering.
3. To motivate the client.	3. Discuss objectives of therapy, including those suggested by the clients.

4. To decrease stuttering symptoms.

4. Describe visual aspects of clients' stuttering. Eliminate some of the objectionable visual aspects by using negative practice. Control blocks by using soft contacts, cancellations and pullouts.

The following objectives and procedures were used with a university-aged client who had pitch-breaks. His friends called him "Squeaky." He seemed anxious to improve his voice and had referred himself to the clinic for therapy.

Objectives	Procedures
1. To determine habitual and optimum pitch levels.	1. Use Fairbank's Method.
2. To determine auditory acuity.	2. Administer sweep hearing test.
3. To determine ability to hear differences in pitch.	3. Administer parts of the Seashore Test of Musical Ability.
4. To determine the possibility of organic causes.	4. Refer client to appropriate medical specialists. (Consult supervisor.)
5. To improve auditory discrimination between pitch levels.	5. Practice discrimination of pitch levels.
6. To establish a lower pitch level.	6. Use optimum pitch level when phonating vowels, reading phrases and sentences, and when conversing. Read and talk with little if any vocal variety.
7. To use variety in pitch without pitch brakes, during conversation.	7. Use optimum pitch level and vocal variety when reading and talking.

PROCEDURES THAT ARE CHALLENGING

If a therapist uses procedures that are too difficult, the client becomes discouraged; and if she uses those that are too easy, not much is accomplished. It is often hard to make decisions concerning procedures that are challenging when clients have complex speech problems that involve combinations of voice, articulation, stuttering and language problems or when the interests and abilities of clients in a group are varied.

A therapist who was helping six college-aged clients from Spanish-speaking countries used the following objectives and procedures:

Objectives	Procedures
1. To improve ability to understand conversational American English.	1. Read short articles from popular magazines. Explain common idioms and slang expressions. Converse with American students.
2. To improve ability to use the inflections and stress patterns of American English.	2. Read marked sentences and paragraphs.
3. To improve ability to hear the following sounds of American	3. Isolate, identify and discriminate the substituted sounds and the

English that are not produced by the clients: [w], [ð], [h] and [ʃ].

acceptable sounds.

4. To improve ability to produce the sounds of American English that are not produced acceptably by the clients.

4. Produce acceptable sounds in isolation, nonsense syllables, words and sentences.

5. To improve ability to use American English in conversation.

5. Study the basic rules of English grammer. Read modern plays. Present short speeches to entertain, to inform and to persuade listeners. Take part in discussions of controversial subjects.

A therapist was giving speech and language therapy to three five-year-old girls in a residential program. They had severe hearing losses and had recently been fitted with hearing aids. She used objectives and procedures similar to these:

Objectives

1. To increase awareness of self.

2. To improve ability to recognize the names of objects and actions.

Procedures

1. Recognize and identify parts of the body.

2. Learn the names of objects and actions used in washing hands, dressing, eating, playing, etc., as the activities are performed. Learn the names of colors. Follow simple directions. Listen to simple stories.

A therapist listed these objectives on a weekly speech and language therapy plan for four adult aphasic clients whose interests and abilities were varied:

Bob: To increase length of attention span and begin to develop an interest in oral communication.

Dorothy: To improve ability to follow instructions and to encourage attempts at verbalization.

Keith: To improve production of [b] and [d] sounds.

Frank: To use a slower rate and a decreased loudness level when speaking.

If you want to improve your ability to formulate objectives and to use procedures that are related to the client's problems, focused and challenging, follow some of these suggestions:

Suggestions for Improving Skill in Using Procedures

1. Compile a list of procedures for use in indirect therapy with delayed speech clients after consulting references such as these:

BACKUS, O., AND BEASLEY, J.: *Speech Therapy with Children.* Boston, Houghton, 1951.

CYPREANSON, L., WILEY, J., AND LAASE, L.: *Speech Development,*

Improvement and Correction. New York, Ronald, 1959.

Low and others: *J Speech Hearing Dis,* Nov., 1959.

MECHAM, M.: Developmental schedules of oral-aural language as an aid to the teacher of the mentally retarded. *Ment Retard,* Dec., 1963, 359-369.

PLOTKIN, W.: *J Speech Hearing Dis,* Feb., 1959.

SMITH, J.: Group language development for educable mental retardates. *Exceptional Child,* 2:29, 1962.

2. Ask yourself the following questions as you observe five therapy sessions:

What procedures were used? Why were they used? What were the apparent assumptions of the therapist? On what information were the procedures based? And what were the results of using the procedures?

Ask yourself somewhat the same questions as you watch some of the following films:

Title: *Speech of Stutterers Before and After Treatment*

Distributor: Audio-Visual Service

              Westbrook Hall

              University of Minnesota

              Minneapolis 14, Minnesota

Title: *Teaching Speech and Language: The McGinnis*

              Association Method

Distributor: Audio-Visual Aids Library

              Pennsylvania State University

              University Park, Pennsylvania

Titles: *Counseling the Adult Stutterer*

        Group Therapy for Aphasia

        Therapy for the Adult Stutterer

Distributor: Bureau of Audio-Visual Instruction

              1312 West Johnson Street

              Madison 6, Wisconsin

3. Use traditional procedures with one group of articulation clients and procedures based on the sensorimotor method with another group of articulation clients. (See McDonald, E.: *Articulation Testing and Treatment: A Sensory-Motor Approach.* 3020 Chartiers Avenue, Pittsburgh, Pennsylvania, Stanwix Housse, Inc.) Compare the results. To what extent do you believe that the results were influenced by differences in the groups of clients

and your training in the use of the two types of procedures?

4. Present one of your stuttering clients to a group of therapists by following some of the suggestions given in Johnson, W., and others: *Speech Handicapped School Children.* New York, Harper, pp. 532-541. Base your discussion of the procedures that you plan to use with the client upon material found in sources similar to these:

CHAPMAN, M.: *Group Therapy for Those Who Stutter.* Minneapolis, Burgess.

JOHNSON, W.: *The Semantics of Stuttering.* Iowa Tapes for Teaching, Iowa City, Iowa, Bureau of Audio-Visual Instruction, State University of Iowa.

LUPER, H., AND MULDER: *Stuttering: Therapy for Children.* Englewood Cliffs, Prentice-Hall.

New Hope for Stutterers (film). Iowa City, Iowa, Bureau of Audio-Visual Instruction, State University of Iowa.

On Stuttering and Its Treatment (a bulletin). 152 Lombardy Road, Memphis, Tennessee, Speech Foundation of America.

ROBINSON, F.: *Introduction to Stuttering.* Englewood Cliffs, Prentice-Hall, 1964.

(Also see "Suggestions for Increasing Knowledge of the Problem," Chapter I.)

5. List the objectives and procedures you plan to use with one of your clients this semester after consulting references similar to those listed below. Give special consideration to the unique aspects of the client's problem.

BLACK, J.: *American Speech for Foreign Students.* Springfield, Thomas.

Foundation of Speech Pathology Series (14 books). Englewood Cliffs, Prentice-Hall.

HANLEY, T.: *Developing Vocal Skills.* New York, Holt, 1962.

HARRIS, G.: *Language for the Preschool Deaf Child.* New York, Grune, 1963.

KARLIN, I., DARLIN, D., AND GURREN, L.: *Development and Disorders of Speech in Childhood.* Springfield, Thomas, 1964.

MASON, S.: *Signs, Signals and Symbols.* Springfield, Thomas, 1963.

SCHUELL, H., JENKINS, J., AND JIMENEZ-PABON, E.: *Aphasia in Adults.* New York, Harper, 1963.

MECHAM, M., and others: *Speech Therapy in Cerebral Palsy.* Springfield, Thomas, 1960.

SNIDECOR, J.: *Speech Rehabilitation of the Laryngectomized.* Springfield, Thomas, 1962.

SPRIESTERSBACH, D., AND SHERMAN, D.: *Cleft Palate and Communication Problems.* New York, Academic Press, 1964.

STRANG, R.: *Hearing Therapy for Children.* New York, Grune, 1955.

STRAUSS, A., AND LEHTINEN, L.: *Psychopathology and Education of the Brain Injured Child.* New York, Grune.

WEST, R., ANSBERRY, M., AND CARR, A.: *The Rehabilitation of Speech.* New York, Harper, 1957.

(Also see "Suggestions for Increasing Knowledge of the Problem," Chapter I.)

6. The following results of articulation testing were obtained from two functional articulation clients each eight years old. Assuming that you decided to use individual direct phoneme-centered therapy, which sound or sounds would you stress first in therapy? Why?

FIRST CLIENT

Omissions	Substitutions
θ (M,F)	w/r (I,M)
r (F)	h/l (I)
ʃ (F)	
	d/θ (I)
tʃ (M,F)	b/ð (M,F)
	d/z (I)
	t/ʃ (I)
	h/j (I)
	t/tʃ (I)
	d/dʒ (I,M)

r
l } Omitted in blends
s

Produced [j] following stimulation.

SECOND CLIENT

Omissions	Substitutions	Distortions
s (M,F)	h/s (I)	v (M)
ʃ (M)	t/k (M)	θ (F)
r (M)	s/ʃ	
	d/dʒ (M)	
	h/f (I,M)	
	t/f (F)	
	d/g (I)	
	t/tʃ (M)	
	h/ʃ (M)	
	b/v (I)	

Produced [v, f and θ] following stimulation.

7. Discuss with your colleagues which of the following eight-year-old functional articulation clients you would place in the same group?

KENNETH

Omissions	Substitutions	Distortions
ʃ (I)	w/r (I)	r (M)
tʃ (F)	s/ʃ (I)	ʃ (M)
r ⎫	l/j (I)	ʒ (M)
s ⎬ Omitted in blends	d/tʃ (I,M)	dʒ (M)
l ⎭	d/dʒ (I)	

Kenneth was not promoted to fourth grade and has frequent temper tantrums. He does not withdraw from speaking situations, but he is, in fact, rather talkative.

RAYMOND

Omissions	Substitutions	Distortions
r (F)	w/r (I,M)	tʃ (I)
ð (M,F)	f/v (I)	
s (F)	t/θ (I,M,F)	
ʃ (M)	s/z (I)	
h (I,M)		
j (I)		
r ⎫		
s ⎬ Omitted in blends		
l ⎭		

Raymond relates well with his teachers and peers, but he does not like school and he has a tendency to withdraw from speaking situations. His school marks are average

MIKE

Substitutions

p/f
b/v
t/θ
d/ð
tʃ/s
dʒ/ʒ

Mike produced his error sounds following stimulation.
He was cooperative during the testing, but somewhat shy. His vocabulary and motor coordination seem to be above average. He is fond of active games.

SALLY

Omissions	Substitutions
r (M,F)	t/k (I,M)
l (I,M,F)	d/g (M)
	b/g (F)
	d/ð
	d/z
	s/ʃ
	s/tʃ

SARAH

Omissions	Substitutions	Distortions
j (I)	w/r (I)	z
	s/dʒ (F)	
	b/f (I,M,F)	
	b/v (I,M,F)	
	d/ð (M)	
	θ/s (I,F)	
	z, t or θ/ʃ	
	s/tʃ	

Sally and Sarah are twins. They enjoy school and their marks are above average. Sally seems to talk much more than Sarah.

8. List appropriate objections and procedures for a semester of speech therapy for one of the clients whose diagnostic evaluations are summarized below:

First Client

Helen started receiving speech therapy in kindergarten. At the present time she is eight years old and in the third grade. Her brother Joseph, who is one year older than she, also has a speech problem. Her early physical development was normal and she has good motor coordination. She does, however, have frequent ear infections. She likes spelling but is having difficulty with arithmetic. According to Mrs. Brown, Helen and Joseph quarrel frequently. Joseph has a tendency to domineer Helen. Helen is rather quiet, bites her nails and twists her hair, but both children are headstrong.

An examination of the oral speech mechanism revealed essentially normal oral structures. It was impossible to initiate a gag reflex. The following consonant substitutions were recorded: w/r, ʃ/tʃ and ʃ/s. She misarticulated several vowels, used substandard grammar and possessed a breathy voice. Her hearing was normal according to an audiometric screening test of the frequencies 500, 1000, 2000, 4000, and 8000 cycles per second at a sensation level of 15 decibels. On the Peabody Picture Vocabulary Test, Form A, her IQ was 86.

Second Client

Jane Bacon had a stroke last year which affected her right side. She is easily frustrated and cries frequently, especially when listeners cannot understand her. She enjoys watching television and frequently walks to the neighborhood grocery store. She becomes upset when she tries to read a newspaper. Eisenson's **Examining for Aphasia** was administered with the following results:

Mrs. Bacon identified the common objects, pictures, colors, forms, numbers, letters and words either by naming them or by pointing to them. Responses to the printed sentences were obtained only by pointing. She recognized sounds, identified body parts and recognized objects placed in her hands. No responses were obtained in verbal or reading comprehension.

She was not able to answer oral questions or the questions relating to the paragraphs read to her, even when given alternate responses. She performed the pretended actions and the imitation tasks satisfactorily. She was able to count to twenty, recite the alphabet, name the days of the weeks and the months of the year. She had difficulty in writing and in wording finding.

Third Client

NAME:
Mark Day

DATE OF INTERVIEW:
February 24, 1966
INFORMANTS:
Mrs. Harris, foster mother, and
Mrs. Shade, social worker

COMPLAINT: Mark's foster mother reported, "He just doesn't pronounce his letters like he should."

HISTORY OF SPEECH DEFECT: Mark's speech problem was present at the time of placement in a foster home on January 22, 1965. Mrs. Shade stated that Mark has received no professional help for his speech problem. During this time Mrs. Harris has tried to show Mark where to put his tongue for certain sounds and how to make them. Mrs. Harris praises Mark when he corrects himself, but if he cannot say the word in question correctly she drops it. She has noticed that Mark can now say the (k) and (d) correctly, especially in the initial position of a word. The social worker agreed that Mark's speech has improved. She believes that Mark and his younger sister find a certain sense of security in using speech which only they can understand. It has been a bond that included only the two of them. Mrs. Harris reported that Mark's speech pattern is pretty consistent, but when talking faster he has more trouble. The foster mother knows of no one who has made any unpleasant comments concerning his speech and she added that both Mark and his sister like to talk.

DEVELOPMENTAL HISTORY: There is no information about Mark's early history. His birth date is May 18, 1958. Mark's own mother is now a patient at a mental institution.

MEDICAL HISTORY: Mark has had only an occasional cold since living with Mrs. Harris. His hearing and vision were checked at school this fall and no impariments were found.

DEVELOPMENT: During the interview Mark's physical behavior was observed and appeared to be within the established norms for seven year olds. He gave his exact age and birth date and talked about his birthday party.

He was able to write the numbers 1 to 20. The size, base line, spacing and method of execution were typical for a seven-year-old.

He was unable to write his name with his left hand, which supports the observation that his right hand has assumed dominance.

MOTOR COORDINATION: Mark has good gross and fine motor coordination and control. He was able to walk a straight line, balance on one foot and touch his nose with the tip of his finger.

RESULTS OF THE PHOTO ARTICULATION TEST: Mark seemed to be very alert and inquisitive, identifying all the items in the test. His vowel sounds were good. He used many glottal stops in the middle of multisyllabic words in the test and in his conversational speech. His errors were as follows:

Omissions	*Substitutions*
s (I)	θ/z (M)
$\int$ (F)	ts/$\int$ (I)
t$\int$ (F)	n/d (M)
t (F)	w/l (I,M)
	s/θ (I,F)
	w/r (I,M)
	t/k (F)

A glottal was substituted for the following sounds in the medial position: [s, t$\int$, d$_3$, θ and p].

Communicative speech was moderately intelligible when the context was known, although his rapid rate combined with his articulation errors, hindered intelligibility. When the context was unfamiliar to the examiner it was very difficult to understand his speech.

ORAL PERIPHERAL EXAMINATION: An oral peripheral examition was administered to Mark. The size and shape of the oral peripheral structures were normal, with class of occlusion being neutrocclusion.

The motility of the structure was good. It is therefore the belief of the examiner that there is nothing in the oral pheripheral mechanism that would interfere with the production of speech.

HEARING EVALUATION: An audiometric sweep examination at 15 decibels was administered. He responded to all frequencies presented.

Chapter V

USING METHODS AND TECHNIQUES

T HERE ARE, PERHAPS, hundreds of methods and techniques that may be used by speech therapists when working with clients. They are the specific means by which therapists help clients attain their objectives. Some representative methods and techniques are described in this chapter, and several sources of others are given in the suggestions at the close of the chapter.

Skilled therapists utilize methods and techniques that are related to the procedures used, they use others after giving the first ones an adequate trial, and they explain them clearly.

METHODS THAT ARE RELATED TO PROCEDURES

Methods and techniques should be related to the specific procedures used with individual clients; however, they are described here by grouping them according to basic procedures that may be used with many clients. The basic procedures are: procedures to modify the client's attitude; exercises to relax the body and to improve the action of the articulators; ear training procedures, production of acceptable speech in simple contexts; and carry-over procedures.

A therapist often modifies a client's attitude toward his speech and toward therapy by creating a desirable atmosphere (see Chapter III, "Creating an Atmosphere"), providing interesting materials and equipment (see Chapter IV, "Using Materials and Equipment") and providing enjoyable speaking experiences (see Chapter VII, "Planning and Reporting Therapy Sessions"). She may also ask questions and provide clear explanations, use the tape recorder and have the client keep records and prepare his own assignments.

Many stutterers seem critical of their own speech and are sometimes helped by a therapist who asks meaningful questions, such as, "During the few moments before you had your most severe block today, what were you thinking?" Some members of one group answered, "I hope I don't stutter," "What will she think of me?", "If I talk fast maybe I won't stutter," "If I stutter, so what; stuttering is no tragedy," and "Perhaps I'll stutter, perhaps I won't; either way I'll talk the best I can." Members of the group discussed the answers, and each client decided what he would say to himself the next time he seemed about to stutter. During one of the first sessions held, the therapist had asked members of the group to draw a line graph representing the changes that had taken place in the severity of their stuttering. Along the abscissa they placed "preschool," "kindergarten," "first grade," "second grade," etc., and along the ordinate numbers representing different levels of severity of stuttering. After the graphs were completed the therapist asked questions such as, "When do you believe your stuttering was most severe?" "Why?" "What factors seemed to be present during the year when your stuttering was least severe?" etc. The questions seemed to encourage them to study their problems more objectively and to become more interested in therapy.

A therapist carefully explained an assignment to a group of

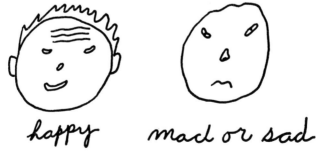

Self-portraits drawn by an eight-year-old stutterer to indicate how he felt before he listened to a tape recording of his speech and after he listened to the tape.

high school articulation clients. She explained why she was giving the assignment and what she hoped the clients would accomplish as a result of performing the assignment.

The tape recorder may be used to help modify the client's attitude toward his speech; however, some precautions seem necessary. (See Chapter VI, "Using Materials and Equipment," for a more complete discussion of the use of tape recorders in therapy.) Most clients are surprised when they hear their voices on tape for the first time. The therapist should explain to older clients, before playing the tapes, that each client hears his own voice by bone conduction; vibrations transmitted through the bones of his head, as well as by air conduction, vibrations transmitted through the air to his ears. He is hearing a different sound than his listeners are hearing and a different sound than the tape recorder is picking up. Some listeners are more sensitive to the high pitches of his voice than are others, and some recorders too, may record certain elements of his voice differently than other recorders. Thus, his voice will probably sound different than he thinks it should when he hears it and it may not even sound as some of his listeners think it does. After playing the recording the therapist may wish to have listeners comment on the naturalness of the recording.

Some recorders are not sensitive to certain types of vocal qualities or lisps. Many therapists record a client's voice, especially one whose problem is mild, at the close of a therapy session and listen to it before the client's next session. If the recording does not adequately portray the client's defect they will not play the recording because they do not wish the client to believe that his speech is normal. Perhaps they will make another recording, setting the tone and/or the intensity controls differently from the settings for the first recording. This may help obtain a recording that is more adequate for their purposes. A different situation is encountered when a client has a very severe speech problem, because listening to a recording may intensify his feeling of hopelessness about his speech. Many therapists record a severe stutterer's speech or a cleft palate client's speech at the close of a therapy session and do not play it back for a few weeks until a second recording is made which shows some improvement.

A therapist helps a client modify his attitude, not only by asking questions, providing explanations and using tape recordings, but also by having him keep records and prepare his own assignments.

One therapist had each client of an eight-year-old articulation group draw a speech rocket in his speech notebook. He listed the following stages that were necessary to fire the rocket and kept a record of the stages he had completed:

> I hear my sound in words;
> I hear when my sound is correct;
> I say my sound correctly by itself;
> I say my sound in words;
> I say my sound when I read;
> I say my sound when I talk.

Another therapist had a group of similar clients draw a living room of a house and the operating and recovery room of a hospital. A small envelope was pasted below each picture. The client wrote words on slips of paper and put the slips into the appropriate envelopes. Slips on which words were written that a client articulated acceptably were placed in the living room envelope. Words that were never produced acceptably were placed in the operating room envelope, and words that were sometimes articulated acceptably were placed in the recovery room envelope.

Members of a group of high school stutterers took turns constructing assignments for all the clients in the group. Each client seemed interested in planning a unique assignment that helped accomplish the objectives the group had set up, and each diligently carried out the assignments.

Many authorities present excellent suggestions and exercises for relaxing the client's body and for improving the action of his articulators. (See some of the references listed at the close of the chapter.) Many therapists believe that these exercises are more beneficial when combined with the production of speech sounds; however, sometimes it seems necessary to concentrate for a period of time upon improving the client's ability to relax or the action of one of his articulators.

A therapist who was working with a college-aged client whose functional hypernasal voice quality had improved very little during one semester of therapy decided to concentrate upon relaxation exercises and exercises to improve velopharyngeal closure. She found that he seemed to be able to relax his throat when performing yawning exercises, especially when he did not complete the yawn.

She had him read short prose selections using increased jaw and lip movements, after explaining to him that the movements of the muscles of the soft palate became more energetic when he used more energetic movement of the jaw and lips. She lowered the back of his tongue with a tongue depressor as he produced some of the low front vowels, in order for him to get the feeling of the lowered position. She had him hold a small mirror under his nose as he produced one of his most nasal vowels. He tried to decrease the amount of clouding of the mirror with each production of the sound. She placed some confetti on a note card he held under his nose and on a note card he held close to his mouth and instructed him to blow the confetti off the upper note card and then off the lower note card. He also became more aware of the action of his soft palate and better able to control the action by pretending to swallow a large piece of candy, by holding his lips closed, filling his mouth and cheeks with breath and releasing the breath through his nose without opening his lips, by producing [æ] and following it with another [æ] pitched an octave higher than the first and by repeating [ʌŋ, a].

Another therapist who was planning to use direct therapy with some cerebral palsied clients who had articulation problems listed the following techniques for helping a client learn to elevate the tip of his tongue. She arranged them according to difficulty, listing first those that would help a client who had little difficulty in elevating the tip of his tongue. After reading the reports of the diagnostic evaluations which indicated that all of the clients could elevate the posterior portion of their tongues, she determined which of the techniques to start using with each client. If the technique chosen was too difficult, she chose a more appropriate one.

1. Client produces one of the sounds requiring elevation of the tip of the tongue, following strong auditory stimulation by the therapist.

2. Client produces one of the above sounds, following observation of therapist in a mirror or an explanation by therapist of a diagram of the articulators, and/or the therapist touches the client's upper alveolar ridge with a tongue blade.

3. Client opens mouth and as he lowers his head, closes his mouth and lifts his tongue.

4. Client attempts to remove peanut butter from upper lips or removes it from upper alveolar ridge, or therapist applies a small wet piece of paper to the tip of the client's tongue and/or the therapist lifts the tongue tip with a tongue blade.

5. Therapist depresses client's tongue tip with a tongue blade and the client resists the movement, or therapist pushes the client's head backward and he resists the movement.

She found that all of the clients except one were able to perform the movement after a few of the techniques had been usd for approximately ten minutes each day for three weeks. The other client learned to produce approximations of the sounds being stressed with the blade rather than the tip of his tongue.

Some ear training methods are described in Chapter VI, "Using Materials and Equipment." Sources of others methods are given in the suggestions at the close of the chapter and a few are described in the next two paragraphs.

A therapist who used indirect therapy with a small group of young articulation clients told the story of *The Gingerbread Boy* the day after the children had a party at which ginger cookies in the shape of the Gingerbread Boy had been served. She said, "This little boy hasn't learned to say his name the way adults say it. When he says dingerbread rather than gingerbread shake your heads." The children listened attentively to the story and shook their heads when the word "gingerbread" was misarticulated. On Halloween she said that she was going to talk like a ghost and that they were to do what the ghost told them to do. She gave directions such as, "Jump on one foot," producing each sound of the words in the sentence separately (in isolation).

A therapist, who was administering direct voice therapy to three college-aged clients with harsh voices, had them read paired sentences. One sentence of the pair contained many words with front vowels in the initial position. The other sentence contained words beginning with consonants. The therapist also had the clients produce [æ] when assuming various head postures. She helped them decide when the sound was produced with the least harshness. They also read sentences before and after taking throat relaxation exercises. The clients soon learned to discriminate between harsh and non-harsh vocal qualities.

Perhaps the most difficult procedure in speech therapy is the production of acceptable speech in simple contexts. A therapist who is giving direct therapy to a group of clients who have hypernasal voice qualities and monotony of pitch, and another group with lateral emissions of sibilants, is very pleased when the clients can produce even one oral vowel and one phrase with variety in pitch or one sibilant sound that is produced with forward emission.

Many therapists use auditory stimulation, phonetic placement and moto-kinesthetic methods or a combination of these methods when teaching production of acceptable speech in simple contexts. Some therapists use other methods such as babbling, chewing and negative practice.

A therapist who was giving direct therapy to a group of high school aged clients who had hypernasal voice quality and monotomy of pitch used the following techniques before all members of the group were able to produce acceptable speech in simple contexts:

1. Combine [h] with open vowels. Exaggerate jaw movement;

2. Whisper open vowels, then produce them with voice;

3. Sing and speak combinations of nonsense syllables such as [ba, bi, bo, zi, zu, za];

4. Hum [m] and direct the breath stream toward the lips, then open the lips and form [a];

5. Produce monosyllabic words containing nasals by separating the nasal from the rest of word. Use the fingers to feel vibrations on the top of the head when the nasal is produced and on the cheeks when the rest of the word is produced;

6. Prolong the nasals when reading short lines of poetry;

7. Count from one to ten starting with a low pitch and raising the pitch as each number is said. Repeat, starting with a high pitch;

8. Use double inflections when repeating vowels, nonsense syllables, words and phrases;

9. Read short sentences using a sudden hard pressure of the abdominal muscles as each breath is exhaled;

10. Read a list of famous quotations, first using a monotonous pitch, then using several steps, then many upward inflections, then many downward inflections and then many double inflections. Finally read the quotations, trying to communicate the meaning.

This therapist used the following techniques with a group of nine-year-old clients who emitted [s] laterally:

1. Present ear training exercises and auditory stimulation using amplification;

2. Use a soda straw held vertically at the level of the top surface of the client's lower lip to determine the place of emission of air. Produce [s] and move the straw until the sound vibrates through the straw. Place the straw at the midline of the lips and, after blowing into the straw a few times, attempt to produce an acceptable [s];

3. Relax the lips and jaw. Keep the teeth slightly open and produce [s] as a sigh is exhaled;

4. Prolong a whispered [hi], gradually open mouth and then gradually close mouth. The [hi] should change to an acceptable [s];

5. Moisten the center of the lower lip so that the flow of air may be felt here. Produce [p] followed by a prolonged [s] and [t];

6. Place tongue in the position for [t]. Open mouth and drop the tip of the tongue away from the upper alveolar ridge and send air through the opening or produce a series of rapid evenly spaced [t] sounds and change the last [t] to [s]. Chant [st, st, t] repeatedly, prolonging the [s];

7. Press the midline of the tongue with the edge of a tongue blade. Close the mouth. Smile. Produce [s];

8. Produce the movements that are necessary for an acceptable [s] slowly, one at a time without breath, then with breath. Increase the speed;

9. Therapist produces a series of nonsense syllables. When [s] is produced in a syllable client repeats the syllable;

10. Carry out directions such as: Stand by the window and produce [s] four times; prolong [s] and gradually increase the loudness level; stand on one foot and repeat [s] until you lose your balance;

11. Give facts about an animal and use [sosi] as the name of the animal. Others in the group will guess the true name of the animal;

12. Prolong [s] until a bell is rung, then say the rest of a word that is written on the blackboard;

13. Repeat words said by therapist while you observe movements of the client's articulators in a mirror;

14. Articulate words containing [s]. Say [s] in isolation following production of the words in which [s] was not produced acceptably;

15. Articulate words containing [s]. Articulate each word once with lateral emission of [s] and twice with forward emission.

Therapists who are using indirect therapy also stress acceptable production of speech in simple contexts. A therapist who was using indirect therapy with a group of young hard-of-hearing clients, brought three colorful pictures of BoBo, the clown, to a therapy session. Below is an account of the session:

Therapist: I have here some pictures of BoBo, the clown. He works at the circus. Who will show me some of the funny things that BoBo does? (Jim makes a face, Ralph stands on his head and James turns cartwheels.)

Therapist: That's right, he does many funny things. How many pictures do I have of BoBo? Let's count them.

Clients: One, two, three.
Therapist: Are the hats alike?
Clients: Yes.
Therapist: Are the collars alike?
Clients: Yes.
Therapist: Are the mouths alike?
Clients: No.

Therapist: That's because BoBo is saying different sounds. Here he's saying [a], here [o] and here [u]. Let's play we are BoBo and do and say some funny things. Put your hands on your hips and shake your head and say[a]. Nod your head and say [o] and lean forward and say [u]. (Therapist performs actions and clients perform the actions as therapist points to the appropriate picture.) Sometimes BoBo says [ma, mo, mu]. We'll say that now. (Clients perform the same actions with other nonsense syllables composed of the initial sounds of [w, b and v] and the three vowels.)

Often younger clients enjoy carry-over activities such as telling stories they have heard or original stories, singing songs and participating in creative play. (See Chapter VI, "Using Materials and Equipment.") A four-year-old delayed speech client enjoyed telling a short original story about a dancing pearl, after he had bounced a pearl bead upon a table and adjacent areas of the therapy room floor. A similar client increased his loudness level after taking part in creative play. He was frequently asked to play the part of the giant in *Jack and the Bean Stalk*.

Some older clients who were participating in a residental program organized a speech club, used passwords, greetings and good-byes, telephoned townspeople to thank them for contributions to the program or to invite them to entertainments. They also explained the program to guests and acted as teachers for some of the younger clients by helping them with their speech workbooks and assignments, constructing therapy materials and supervising simple speech drills.

High school and college-aged clients frequently read orally, practice for the speaking experiences they have outside the clinic and perform assignments similar to those given in public speaking classes, in order to make their acceptable speech habitual. Often those who stutter are encouraged to join groups in which speaking is required.

When indirect therapy is used the therapist usually does not interrupt the carry-over activity, but she frequently records or remembers the unacceptable speech used in the activity and uses it as a basis for further activities that stress acceptable speech in simple contexts. When carry-over activities are first used in direct therapy the therapist or members of the group may point out and correct errors immediately after they occur. Later the therapist may prefer to list the errors made and use them in a drill at the close of the session.

METHODS THAT ARE VARIED

Some therapists fail to use other methods and techniques after giving the first ones an adequate trial. One therapist continued to use the same method with a young client with expressive language problems for an entire semester without results. Another therapist tried auditory stimulation with an eight-year-old general American client who misarticulated [a]. After using this method with him for approximately six therapy sessions, the therapist had him lie on a table in the therapy room. He was then able to produce an acceptable [a] and later learned to make this sound acceptably while sitting in a chair. He learned to produce [ar] by using the following techniques.

1. Touch the roof of the mouth with the tongue tip in the area of the soft palate, then the middle of the mouth, above the alvealor ridge and above the central incisors.

2. Widen the tongue and lift it. Spread it so it can be felt against the sides of the teeth.

3. Therapist pulls the corners of the lower lip downward and slightly backward after client starts to phonate [a]. Client elevates the whole tongue and moves the tip slightly back and prolongs [a] until it changes to [ar].

Another therapist found that a cerebral palsied client, eleven years old, improved her articulation when she spoke just above a whisper using a minimum of effort. Relaxation exercises seemed to help this client, especially relaxation of the vocal mechanism, as the client gripped the arms of a chair.

Relaxation exercises also helped an adult aphasic, as did drills in which the client sang the words of a sentence before saying them, closed her eyes when repeating a sentence, prolonged each sound of a sentence, performed amplified ear training exercises and repeated the words of a simple paragraph as the therapist continued to read it. The therapist discovered that a technique that was successful during one therapy session could not be used during another session. In order to help reduce the confusion for the client that resulted from varying the techniques, the order of the type of technique used was kept stable. During some sessions the client continued using one technique for a long period of time without becoming tired or bored, even though it was not successful. The therapist learned to gauge the amount of variation of techniques to suit the client's daily needs, ability and interest.

METHODS THAT ARE CLEARLY EXPLAINED

Skilled therapists carefully explain the methods and techniques clients use. When a therapist uses indirect therapy she gives clear explanations of what the client is to do, but she does not explain the reasons behind the techniques or the theory upon which the technique is based. With younger clients she may need to present one part of an explanation and wait until the clients perform this part of the task before she gives the next part. She may make her explanations clearer by performing the task herself.

When a therapist uses direct therapy she explains why she is using the technique, what it is and how the client is to carry it out. She gives most of these explanations before the client uses the technique. One therapist explained voluntary stuttering to a group of high school stutterers and told them she was having them use it to help them control their stuttering. Another therapist told a similar group that they were to use the technique so that they would lose some of their fear of stuttering. The two groups probably performed the technique differently and with different results because of the differences in the explanations. Some therapists give explanations that are too detailed while others make them too brief. The therapist needs, of course, to consider the abilities of the client, the length of his attention span, his level of receptive language, etc. when giving explanations. Lack of a clear explanation at the appropriate time often wastes valuable therapy time. Some therapists, for example, ask a client to evaluate a tape recording after the recording has been played, rather than before. The recording often has to be replayed before the evaluation can be made.

Therapists have improved their ability to use methods and techniques by following suggestions similar to those listed below.

Suggestions for Improving Skill in Using Methods and Techniques

1. Use some of the diagrams and explanations given in references similar to the following, in order to acquaint a group of adult voice articulation or hard-of-hearing clients with one of the processes of speech or hearing:

HELLER, M.: *Functional Otology.* New York, Springer, 1955.

KAPLAN, H.: *Anatomy and Physiology of Speech.* New York, McGraw, 1960.

SHEARER, W.: *Illustrated Speech Anatomy.* Springfield, Thomas, 1963.

2. When helping a young client with language problems, apply some of the concepts from operant conditioning after reading sources similar to the following:

HOLLAND, A., AND MATTHEWS, J.: Application of teaching machine concepts to speech pathology and audiology. *ASHA,* Jan., 1963, 474-482.

MEDNICK, S.: *Learning.* Englewood Cliffs, Prentice-Hall, 1964. See especially Chapters 3, 4 and 6.

3. Read abstracts of eight research studies in the field of stuttering and modify some of the techniques used in the studies for use in group therapy with high school stutterers.

4. In order to improve the methods you use with one group

of clients, read at least three appropriate journal articles. Consult the *Cumulative Indexes of the Journals of the American Speech and Hearing Association.*

5. Suggest how the therapist who wrote the following two reports might have improved communication with her functional articulation client, eight years old:

> September 23
>> Irene mentioned that she did not like speech class at all. So we went over the purpose of a speech class and added that it can be pleasant and enjoyable.
>
> October 21
>> When Irene was asked if she tried speaking with the new speech rate that she had used when making a recording last week, she responded with a positive remark. The next question asked was if she liked speaking like that and if others noticed it and used it to. She answered in the affirmative.

6. Start a file of useful methods and techniques. Place a description of one method or technique on each index card used. Organize the file according to the basic procedures listed in this chapter or according to a plan that suits your individual needs better than either of these. You may remove cards from the file, attach them to a clipboard and use them when presenting a therapy session, much as a public speaker uses note cards when presenting a speech. You may use your textbooks and many of the references listed at the close of other chapters of this book, as well as references similar to these as sources of the methods and techniques.

ADLER, S.: *The Non-Verbal Child.* Springfield, Thomas, 1964.

AGRANOWITZ, A., AND McKEOWN, M.: *Aphasia Handbook: For Adults and Children.* Springfield, Thomas, 1963.

BARRY, H.: *The Young Aphasic Child.*

BRYNGELSON, B., CHAPMAN, M., AND HANSEN, O.: *Know Yourself: A Workbook for Those Who Stutter.* Minneapolis, Burgess, 1958.

BRYNGELSON, B., AND MIKALSON, E.: *Speech Correction Through Listening.* New York, Scott.

BYRNE, M.: *The Child Speaks, A Speech Improvement Program for Kindergarten and First Grade.* New York, Harper, 1965.

CHAPMAN, M.: *Self-Inventory: Group Therapy for Those Who*

Stutter. Minneapolis, Burgess, 1959.

DECKER, F.: *Progressive Lessons for Language Retraining.* New York, Harper, 1960.

FAIRBANKS, G.: *Practical Voice Practice.* New York, Harper, 1944.

——————: *Voice and Articulation Drillbook.* New York, Harper, 1960.

FIELDS-BENDER: *Voice and Diction.* New York, Macmillan, 1949.

GREGORY, H.: Speech clinic helps the adult stutterer. *Rehab Rec,* Nov.-Dec., 1964.

GORDON, M.: *A Manual for Speech Improvement.* Englewood Cliffs, Prentice-Hall, 1961.

HAWK, S.: *Speech Therapy for the Physically Handicapped.* Stanford, Stanford U P, 1950.

JACOBSON, E.: *Progressive Relaxation.* Chicago, U of Chicago, 1938.

Journal of Verbal Learning and Verbal Behavior. (Contains reports of research in psycholinguistics.) 35 B New Street, Worcester, Massachusetts.

Journals of the American Speech and Hearing Association. 9030 Old Georgetown Road, Washington, D. C. (See *Cumulative Indexes,* 1962.)

KARR, H.: *Developing Your Speaking Voice.* New York, Harper, 1953.

KEPHART, N.: *The Slow Learner in the Classroom.* Columbus, Charles E. Merrill.

LUPER, H., AND MULDER, R.: *Stuttering Therapy for Children.* Englewood Cliffs, Prentice-Hall, 1964.

McGINNIS, M.: *Aphasic Children.* 1537 West 35th Street, Northwest, Washington, D. C., Alexander Graham Bell Association for the Deaf.

MARTIN, B.: *Communicative Aids for the Adult Aphasic.* Springfield, Thomas, 1962.

MECHAM, M.: Developmental schedules of oral-aural language as an aid to the teacher of the mentally retarded. *Ment Retard,* Dec., 1963.

NEMOY, E., AND DAVIS, S.: *The Correction of Defective Consonant Sounds.* Magnolia, Expression.

OJEMANN, R., HAWKINS, A., AND CHOWNING, K.: *A Teaching Program in Human Behavior and Mental Health.* Iowa City, State U of Iowa, 1961. (Several publications.)

SHACTER, H., AND BAUER, W.: *You and Others.* (Health and personal development program—a series of books for elementary schools.)

SHEEHAN, J.: *Scientific Approaches to Stuttering.* New York, Harper, 1966.

Speech Pathology and Therapy (journal). North Circular Road, Neasden, London N.W. 10, Book Centre Ltd.

TAYLOR, G.: *Learning American English.* New York, McGraw.

Treatment of Stuttering in the Schools (pamphlet). Speech Foundation of America.

VAN RIPER, C., AND BUTLER, K.: *Speech in the Elementary Classroom.* New York, Harper, 1955.

Your state or regional Speech and Hearing Association journal or newsletter.

WOLPE, J.: The systematic desensitization treatment of neurosis. *J Nerv Ment Dis,* 1961. (Describes a technique that may be used with stutterers and perhaps other clients.)

ZEDLER, E.: *Listening for Speech Sounds.* New York, Harper, 1955.

7. A therapist who was working with a seven-year-old client with ataxia made the following transcription of a tape-recorded therapy session. Evaluate the methods and techniques she used.

Therapist: Remember, Kent, last week we used the stopwatch and the clock to see how long we could hold the sound.

Kent: Yes.
Therapist: [e].
Kent: [e].

Therapist: You get out of breath if you take too long. O.K.? Now, what are we going to remember? We try to hold this sound? We're going to take a what? A deep breath? Right? O.K. Let's draw a line across here. You take a piece of chalk. O.K. You got it? Let's see if there's anymore chalk. O.K. There isn't. We'll try this [e] sound. This will be our first try, our second, our third and our fourth time. We'll use the second hand of the clock. We need some lines across here. O.K. Now I'll watch the time and after you finish saying it, you'll write it in. O.K.? Now the first sound is what?

Kent: [e].
Therapist: O.K. Now listen. See how long you can hold that sound. O.K.? Get ready, get set, go.

Kent: [e].
Therapist: Good. You held that for twelve seconds. Write a twelve up there. O.K. Let's try [i]. Get ready, get set, go.

Kent: [i].

Therapist: Oh, you held that for about six seconds.

Kent: Do I put it here?

Therapist: No, you put it by the [i]. O.K. Now the [ai] sound. Get ready, get set, go.

Therapist: How come, you think, you were able to make that sound so long? Did you take a deep breath? Or did your breath go through your nose? Did the air come out your nose or your mouth?

Kent: Out of my nose.

Therapist: You think the air came out of your nose? Come over here, Kent. Put your hand up in front of your mouth and your nose. Now say [o].

Kent: [o].

Therapist: Where is the air coming from?

Kent: From my mouth.

Therapist: Right, what's our last sound? [e, i, ai, o] What's our last sound?

Kent: [ju].

Therapist: [ju]. Get ready, get set, go.

Kent: [ju].

Therapist: Five seconds. You didn't hold that one very much. If you're going to sit on the chair remember to use your good posture for speech. Head up. Chest in. Your tummy in, I mean. Let's see if you can beat me on the [o] sound. Get ready, get set, go. [o].

Kent: [o].

Therapist: Ten seconds on the [o] sound. What other sounds did we work on last time?

Kent: I don't know.

Therapist: What's this sound? (Therapist knocks on the table.) The woodpecker sound. Can you make that sound? (Kent knocks on the table.) Can you make that sound for me on our lips and in our mouth?

Kent: [d, d].

Therapist: And, what's the [t, t, t] sound?

Kent: The clock sound.

Therapist: Right: Our friend, the clock. Can you think of some words that have the woodpecker sound in them? You're looking at your book, aren't you?

Kent: No, I ain't.

Therapist: Can you think of others?

Kent: No.

Therapist: Let's think of some with the clock sound?

Kent: Train.

Therapist: Right. Where do you shoot a bow and arrow? or when something rings? at home and you answer it?

Kent: Telephone.

Therapist: Fine. Now, I'm going to give you some numbers, Kent, and I want to see if you can repeat them back to me. They get longer and longer and longer. One, two.

Kent: One, two, buckle my shoe. Three, four, shut the door.

Therapist: Maybe you didn't understand me. I'm going to say some numbers and you say them back to me. Ready? One, two.

Kent: One, two, buckle my shoe.

Therapist: When I say "one, two" I want to see if you can say "one, two," too. I'll say "one, two."

Kent: One, two.

(Therapist and Kent continue with the auditory memory span for digits test.)

Therapist: Now, I'd like you to read a story for me.

8. A therapist made the following notes as she read the diagnostic folder of Dotty Evans, the client she had been assigned for the semester. What methods, techniques and materials would be appropriate for use, in your opinion, with Dotty?

Dotty, severe motor-speech difficulty.

CA—four year eight months.

Meningitis when she was two years one month old. For six weeks after returning from the hospital had nightmares every night.

Has an imaginary friend.

Is shy and afraid of strange situations.

Average intelligence.

Adequate inner and receptive language.

During articultaion testing, produced only vowels and a

few initial consonants. Did not produce medial or final consonants. Did not produce medial or final consonants following strong stimulation.

Below average, perhaps inferior, oral motor coordination.

Chapter VI

USING MATERIALS AND EQUIPMENT

In order to motivate and interest the client, materials and equipment should be sufficiently varied, original, adequately placed and fully used. Therapists sometimes use the same

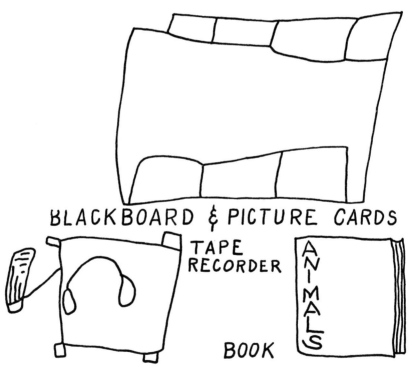

Drawn in answer to the question, "What materials do we use in speech class?" by a nine-year-old client who was attending an EMH class.

materials and equipment session after session; they often use materials and equipment commonly used by other therapists; they fail to realize the importance of the placement of materials and equipment; and do not use those they provide intensively.

MATERIALS THAT ARE SUFFICIENTLY VARIED

Skilled therapists often use a variety of materials that appeal to the client's senses, especially when the use of such materials does not confuse the client. A therapist who conducted beginning auditory training sessions with four children who had moderate hearing losses used the following materials during five consecutive therapy sessions: sounds in the therapy room; noisemakers; bongo drums; bells; a violin; rhythm band instruments; records of Sousa marches; and a reading of Poe's "The Bells." These materials were used with discriminative, rhythmic and creative exercises. The exercises included listening activities, calisthenics, Indian dances, movement to music while pretending to be rag mops, popcorn popping, etc., keeping time with the recordings and marching. The clients enjoyed using the materials, became more interested in sounds and improved their auditory discrimination. One cerebral palsied client who had previously shown little interest in therapy actively participated in the sessions and during some sessions enjoyed operating the record player.

Another therapist used a variety of oral reading materials in the carry-over stage of articulation therapy with seven high school aged clients. The clients read short editorials which they brought to the therapy session and told why they agreed or disagreed with the editor. Later, two of the editorials were used as the basis for group discussions. At another time each client brought in the script of a modern play. He used acceptable articulation when presenting a synopsis of the play. When reading a scene involving two characters, he used acceptable articulation as he read one character's lines and unacceptable articulation when reading the other character's lines. Later, the therapist brought in scripts of one of Noel Coward's plays and the clients read the parts with precise British articulation. She also cut articles entitled "You Be The Judge" from a popular magazine. The clients read these articles and discussed orally what decision the judge should have given. Another therapist obtained free story books from The Dairy Council. Each young articulation client in a group was given a book. They were asked to turn the pages of their book as the therapist read the story. The therapist did not realize how difficult this would be for these clients. She asked the clients to take their books and have their mothers or fathers finish the story, because the story was constantly interrupted by remarks such as, "Where is that picture?" "Show me," "I can't find it," etc. Perhaps if she had been more skillful or more patient she could have taught the clients to turn the pages of the books. She thought she had been more successful during a session with stutterers when she had them read an article on attitudes of handicapped persons toward their problems. Each client read the article, prolonging the first sound of the words on which he expected to stutter. The activity seemed to help modify the client's speech as well as their attitudes.

Therapists have effectively used such visual aids as flannel boards, wall charts and filmstrips. A therapist who had trouble eliciting speech from a fourteen-year-old mentally retarded client showed him a filmstrip about boats. The strip helped focus his attention and encouraged him to talk of his experiences with his father's motor boat. She discovered that a small group of cerebral palsied clients accomplished more when she remembered to bring each client a mirror to use when practicising tongue exercises than when she failed to bring the mirrors. They were also interested in using the large laminated wood spinner board which she had a carpenter construct so that it could be hung on the wall and used with a variety of materials.

A therapist decided to use the opaque-projector to show pictures illustrating "T'was the Night Before Christmas" as a recording of the poem was played to a group of young clients with delayed speech. The boys in the group were much more interested in looking at the projector and in trying to find out how it worked than in the pictures or the poem. The therapist remembered how interested a group of older boys had been in a unit on simple machines and another group in a unit on the planets, and decided to try to adapt material from science for use in indirect speech therapy.

Therapists not only provide a variety of auditory and visual materials, but also material that has tactile and/or kinesthetic appeal. Three young hard-of-hearing clients soon learned the meaning of the word "kitty" while playing with and feeding a black kitten. A delayed speech client enjoyed observing and talking about two small turtles. A four-year-old delayed speech client observed a bulldozer digging a basement and later used several short sentences as he played with a toy bulldozer in the sandbox. A twelve-year-old mentally retarded girl enjoyed setting out and taking care of a geranium.

An experienced therapist thought that she was relying too extensively upon materials and decided to store them for a week. During this time she discovered that often she did not need to use materials and she developed ideas for materials that were more varied and original than those she had been using.

MATERIALS THAT ARE ORIGINAL

Some supervisors insist that therapists construct all of their materials and use many materials that are not commonly used by other therapists. This requirement seems time-consuming and limits the therapist; however, even beginning therapists may be encouraged to experiment with materials. The experimentation often benefits the clients and frequently makes speech therapy more interesting to the therapist.

Therapists may use materials that are easily available but seldom used in therapy, or they may use materials in an original manner. A therapist provided each of the boys in an articulation therapy group with a piece of string approximately twelve inches in length. After a discussion of types of knots, each client tied four knots in his piece of string. Then they took turns producing [s] in isolation for the length of time that it took them to slide their fingers from one knot to the next along the string. The therapist asked each client to take the string home and, after practicing his sound, show some member of his family the string and how well he could produce his sound. She had two younger articulation clients make mobiles out of coat hangers. They used colored string to tie small objects purchased from the dime store to the hangers. On one coat hanger they tied the objects whose names contained the [s] sound and, on the other, those containing the [tʃ] sound. After the clients learned to articulate correctly the names of the articles, they hung the mobiles above the door of the therapy room and repeated the name of one of the articles each time they walked under the mobile.

Another therapist used paper bags effectively. During one session she stood at one end of the therapy room and held a large paper bag. Each client pretended to throw his sound into the bag when producing it in isolation. If the sound was acceptably articulated the therapist made a noise that indicated that the sound had hit the bag. She made another noise to indicate that the sound was not acceptably articulated and had missed the bag. She had a group of young cleft palate clients make Halloween masks from paper bags. Each mask was made with a very large cutout mouth. The clients used crayons to decorate the masks. When the masks were completed the clients put them on and produced vowel sounds, opening their own mouths as widely as the mouths of their masks. At another time three 4-year-old delayed speech clients acted out *The Three Little Kittens* as they operated hand puppets made from small paper bags. The clients stood behind a small screen set up in front of other delayed speech clients and held the puppets above the screen.

Anothr therapist had three older mentally retarded clients construct a portable doll house from four pieces of cardboard. They papered each piece of cardboard on both sides with wallpaper from sample books. The four pieces were put together like a notebook with four large notebook rings. When they played with the house they stood the pieces on end and separated them at right angles to each other in order to form rooms. The rooms had no outer walls. These boys enjoyed constructing the house, furnishing it with samples of carpets, toy furniture from the dime store, etc. and playing with it. Their ability to understand language and to organize and express their thoughts improved during these activities. Other groups of clients constructed garages and space stations, using similar basic materials.

Some therapists use the blackboard in original ways. One had a group of articulation clients write an O on the board when they heard the acceptable production of the sound on which they were working, and an X when they heard the substituted sound. During sessions held after the clients could produce the sound acceptably, the therapist wrote a series of Xs interspersed with O's on the board and the clients produced the indicated sounds as she pointed to each symbol. She left these symbols on the board and used them with other groups, including those who were correcting a sound different from the one the first group was correcting. These symbols were also used when the groups were producing nonsense syllables. At another time she wrote a paragraph loaded with [r] on the board with the [r] sounds underlined. Groups that were correcting this sound and were ready for carry-over read the paragraph in unison. Groups that were correcting another sound read the paragraph, substituting their sound for the [r] sounds. One day she asked third grade clients to pass to the blackboard and draw the back of a house and the front of a house. Then she said, "If I say [ti], which as you know it made with your tongue close to the front of your mouth, point to the front door of the house you have drawn. If I say [ki] point to the back door."

A therapist with some imagination had a cleft palate client with a short attention span make soap carvings. During a few therapy sessions for young delayed speech clients, she provided boxes filled with small pieces of silk, colored lace, pictures from old Christmas cards, etc. to use in making Christmas collages. She asked them questions and encouraged conversation as they chose materials and made the collages. After the collages were finished each child told a story about his picture. The collages were later used to decorate the therapy room. At another time she told these clients a story about the *Speech Bunny*. She wrote letters to each client, praising the client for something he had accomplished in therapy or encouraging him to accomplish more. The letters were signed Your Friend, The Speech Bunny and included a picture of the bunny. Later she used a series of dittoed pictures to encourage each child to tell an original story, and she asked questions about the pictures to encourage reluctant clients to talk.

MATERIALS AND EQUIPMENT THAT ARE ADEQUATELY PLACED AND FULLY USED

Many therapists realize the importance of presenting one material at a time to clients who are distractable and keeping other materials stored until they are ready to use them. Sometimes, however, they fail to realize that the placement of chairs, tables, blackboards, mirrors, etc. may affect the results of therapy.

A therapist who was giving therapy in a large playroom found that clients did not run aimlessly around the room as much during play periods when chairs and tables were moved so that they filled the spaces more adequately. She also discovered that the blackboards and bulletin boards were more usable when they were lowered so that the center of the material placed on them was as the client's eye level.

Many therapists use tape recorders in speech therapy even though the effects of their use have not been investigated adequately. Recordings may be repeated, are permanent, and the client may listen to them independent of simultaneous production. Therapists have discovered, however, that clients vary in their ability to benefit from listening to recordings of their own voices.

Some stutterers benefit from a period of therapy involving the use of tape recordings. (See Davis, D.: *An Exploratory Study of the Use of Tape Recordings in Stuttering Therapy.* Ann Arbor, University Microfilms Inc., Order No. 65-964.) At the present time, a trial period of therapy seems to be the only method available for deciding which stuttering clients will benefit from the intensive use of tape recordings. At the close of the trial period the clients and the therapist should evaluate the effect of the use of the recordings.

In the study mentioned above, clients made and listened to tape recordings of their own oral reading and discussed what they heard with their therapist. In the trial period or during a longer period, therapists may wish to follow procedures similar to those that were used in the study.

Procedure for Listening *Therapy Sessions*	*Time Allotted* *(each week)*
Client reads from a passage 4 consecutive times for 2 minutes each time. Reading is recorded.	8 minutes
He listens to readings just recorded.	8 minutes
He reads from a passage 4 consecutive times for 2 minutes each time. Reading is recorded.	8 minutes
He listens to second recording.	8 minutes
Therapy related to the listening is administered.	28 minutes

Only the therapist and the client were present when the recordings were made. The client held the directional microphone approximately eight inches from his mouth and followed the oral instructions the therapist gave him. The therapist advised him to stutter as much as he wanted to, but in an easy and as relaxed a manner as possible.

The therapists gave the clients the following instructions concerning listening to the tape recordings:

"Please listen carefully to your readings." (The rest of the instructions varied with the lesson plan of the week. The following instructions were given when the client wrote a description of his speech.) "When you have finished listening I'll ask you to write a description of how you sound when you read aloud, especially when you stutter. I'll want you to describe your speech in detail, so listen as carefully as you can and do not talk unless you are asked a question." (Client listens for eight minutes and writes the description.) During other listening therapy sessions he engaged in therapy after the listening— see lesson plans and a description of a lesson below.

Weekly Lesson Plans for Therapy Related to the Recordings

First Week

OBJECTIVE: To encourage the client to express his true attitude toward his speech.

PROCEDURES: He will write a description of how he sounds when he reads, especially when he stutters, and he will describe orally his attitude toward his speech. In order to encourage him to express his true attitude, the therapist will use a client-centered counseling approach. She will accept his feelings and echo them.

Second Week

OBJECTIVE: To encourage the client to develop a more objective attitude toward his speech.

PROCEDURES: Therapist will continue the client-centered approach. Client will define and give examples of an objective attitude. Therapist will supply information when necessary.

Therapist will describe briefly the Berwick study and ask the client if he considers himself a hard listener insofar as his own speech is concerned.

Third Week

OBJECTIVE: To encourage the client to develop his ability to describe his speech.

PROCEDURES: Client will describe his speech. Therapist will encourage him to use concrete descriptive words and to express an objective attitude toward his stuttering.

Fourth Week

OBJECTIVE: To study how the client manages not to say words.

PROCEDURES: Client will tally the number of avoidances and postponements in his recordings, and he and the therapist will discuss their effect on his speech.

He will tally his tense blocks and therapist will encourage him to use less tense blocks in his speaking and reading.

During the last session of the listening therapy the client will write a description of how he sounds when he reads, especially when he stutters.

Description of Second Week Lesson

OBJECTIVE: To encourage the client to develop a more objective attitude toward his speech.

DESCRIPTION OF PROCEDURES: Before the client listened to his recordings, the therapist requested him to listen carefully and told him that after the listening he would be asked to describe his attitude toward his speech. After the listening, the therapist asked the following questions: "How do you feel about your speech?" "What is your attitude toward your speech?" "When you talk to yourself about your speech what do you say?" To encourage the client to express his true attitude the therapist was accepting of his feelings and echoed them. When he remarked, "My speaking is just a waste of words," the therapist replied, "You believe that often you are wasting words when you speak." This procedure was continued for approximately fifteen minutes. (The same procedure had been followed for twenty-eight minutes the preceding week.)

When the client could not give examples of an objective attitude, the therapist asked him to describe the room in which the therapy was being conducted. She asked him to describe it as an impartial observer (a scientist for example) might describe it. She added to his description and suggested that this method could be used when he described or talked about his speech.

Then the therapist explained that Berwick had found an increase in stuttering when a stutterer read facing a front-view photograph of a person he had previously rated as a hard listener. (A person to whom the stutterer felt it was difficult to talk.) There was less increase in stuttering when he read facing a photograph of an easy listener. The therapist then asked, "What effect do you think you have on your own speech? As a listener to your own speech? Do you consider yourself an easy listener? Or a hard one?"

Therapists and clients may wish to use the following scale and the sample descriptions to help them improve the descriptions the client writes or gives orally of his reading and his stuttering:

Scale for Judging Descriptions of Oral Reading and Stuttering

1. Client expresses an entirely objective attitude toward his stuttering; indicates that his stuttering reactions are entirely under his control, applies concrete descriptive words and is fully aware that his remarks express his own opinion.

2. Client expresses a somewhat objective attitude toward his stuttering; indicates that his stuttering reactions are somewhat under his control, applies fairly concrete descriptive words and is somewhat aware that his remarks express his own opinion.

3. Client expresses a neutral attitude toward his stuttering;

does not indicate that his stuttering reactions are under his control, applies few concrete descriptive words and does not indicate that his remarks express his own opinion.

4. Client expresses a somewhat subjective attitude toward his stuttering; indicates that his stuttering reactions are somewhat uncontrollable, applies rather abstract words and is somewhat unaware that his remarks express his own opinion.

5. Client expresses an entirely subjective attitude toward his stuttering; indicates that his stuttering reactions are not under his control, applies abstract words and is entirely unaware that his remarks express his own opinion.

Descriptions Illustrating Three Levels of Adequacy

(Chosen from among those written by the clients at the beginning and at the close of the listening therapy sessions; a rating of *one* represents a most adequate description and a rating of *five* a least adequate description.)

The following description was given a rating of 1.67:

My manner of speech when stuttering can differ three different ways: first of all, the most common way in which I stutter would be the prolongation of the first syllables. The sounds on which this is very noticeable are the F's and S's. The second way, would be stuttering like an ordinary layman would expect a person to stutter; that is, the repetition of sounds. This occurs usually when I am excited and trying to read rapidly. Finally, the last way in which I stutter would be times when I am unable to say anything at all. This happens almost exclusively on the M's at the beginning of phrases and sentences and a few times on other sounds.

The next description was given a rating of 2.67:

How I sound while reading aloud: While reading aloud my voice is fairly normal except when I'm about to stutter. Then I start sliding over words in order to get past the word I think I'll stutter on. In order to avoid stuttering on a word I might skip the first few letters of the word or maybe some of the middle letters. At times when I am about to stutter I might substitute words for words I'll stutter on, and the whole sentence will turn out to be just a waste of words.

The last sample description included here was
given a rating of 4.00:

> My voice sounded the same as it usually does. Whenever
> I got to a block, my throat got tense and the words didn't
> sound normal or as clear as the ones that came out more
> smoothly. Whenever I keep on reading over something my
> throat got more tense and the words sounded worse and
> won't come out.

Therapists often use tape recordings with other types of
clients. One therapist had voice clients listen to tapes they had
made. She asked them questions about the tapes as she played
them. The questions were, of course, difficult to understand and
should have been asked before the tape was played or during
times when the recorder was stopped. Another therapist effectively used tape recordings during several sessions with a nine-
year-old client who had expressive language problems and a
rapid rate of speaking. He evaluated his taped oral reading and
compared it with the choral reading he made with the therapist.
He pretended he was a radio announcer describing two boys
fishing, and at another time that he was calling a friend over
the telephone. He recorded a short story, first using a rapid and
then a slow rate, he talked using slow-motion speech and when
repeating what the therapist said as she continued to talk.

The following suggestions have been designed to help improve your ability to use materials and equipment more
effectively:

Suggestions for Improving Skill in Using
Materials and Equipment

1. Obtain price lists or catalogs from some sources similar to
the following. Which of the advertised educational materials
and equipment would help you most with the clients you now
have?

Council for Exceptional Children, Director of Sales, 1201 16th Street,
Northwest, Washington 6, D. C.

Creative Playthings Inc., P.O. Box 1100, Princeton, New Jersey.

Educational Publishing Corporation, Darien, Connecticut.

Educational Service Inc., Benton Harbor, Michigan.

Educators Progress Service, Randolph, Wisconsin.
Fearon Publishers Inc., 828 Valencia Street, San Francisco, California.
Gaston Manufacturing Co., 234 West Second Street, Cincinnati, Ohio.
Golden Press, Inc., 1 West 39th Street, New York 18, New York.
Milton-Bradley Co., Springfield, Massachusetts.
Model School Supply Co., 1602 Hodiamont Avenue, St. Louis 12, Missouri.
Old King Cole, Inc., Canton, Ohio.
F. A. Owen Publishing Co., Dansville, New York.
W. H. Schafer Manufacturing Co., Inc., Minneapolis, Minnesota.
Therap-Aids, 115 W. Fair Oaks, San Antonio, Texas.
Wood Play, Kemberton, Pennsylvania.

2. Adapt some of the games, activities, etc., found in some children's magazines such as *Highlights, Jack and Jill* and *Humpty-Dumpty,* for use with some of your clients.

3. Construct a form for evaluating speech therapy materials. Use the form to evaluate ten dollars worth of materials purchased from sources similar to these:

Aural-Aids, P.O. Box 5353, Inglewood, California.
Chronicle Guidance Publications, Inc., Moravia, New York.
The Continental Press, Inc., Elizabethtown, Pennsylvania.
Di-Bur Card Games, Box 1184, Pueblo, Colorado.
Expression Co., P.O. Box 11, Magnolia, Massachusetts.
Go-Mo Products, Inc., Box 143, Waterloo, Iowa.
Interstate Printers and Publishers, Danville, Illinois.
King Co., 2414 W. Lawrence Avenue, Chicago 25, Illinois.
Pollywog Publications, 5548 W. Gladys Avenue, Chicago, Illinois.
Selected Creative Communication, Box 703, Santa Anna, California.
Sound Materials, P.O. Box 453, Knoxville, Tennessee.
Stanwix House, Inc., Pittsburgh 4, Pennsylvania.
Charles C Thomas, Springfield, Illinois.
Warnock-Medlin Word Making Cards, P.O. Box 305, Salt Lake City, Utah.
Webster Publishing Co., 1154 Reco Avenue, St. Louis, Missouri.

4. List at least seven ways in which you might use each of the following materials in speech therapy:

> construction paper   ten pipe cleaners
> a newspaper   a game of checkers

5. Order at least two of the following which contain biblio-

graphies of therapy materials:

Boson University, Speech Department: *An Annotated Bibliography of Speech Therapy Materials.*

Chicago Public Schools, Curriculum Department: *Handbook of Speech Therapy.*

Detroit Public Schools: *Speech Therapy Handbook.*

Minneapolis Public Schools: *A Bibliography for Speech Correction.*

Rochester, New York, Public Schools: *Improving Speech.*

6. Read articles similar to the following for suggestions concerning the use of tape recordings with stutterers:

CYPREANSEN, L.: Group therapy for adult stutterers. *J Speech Hearing Dis, 13*:313-319, Dec., 1948.

LEMERT, E., AND VAN RIPER, C.: The use of psychodrama in the treatment of speech defects. *Sociometry,* May, 1944, pp. 190-195.

7. Suppose you have five hundred dollars to spend for records, films and equipment for a new speech clinic serving a variety of clients. Order catalogs or price lists from companies similar to the following and decide what you would purchase with the money:

Children's Music Center, 2858 West Pico, Los Angeles 6, California.

Children's Press Inc., Chicago, Illinois.

Coronet Films, Coronet Building, Chicago 1, Illinois.

Educational Records, 10515 Burbank, North Hollywood, California.

Ekstein Bros., 1907 Beverly, Los Angeles, California.

Electronic Teaching Laboratories, 5034 Wisconsin Avenue, Northwest, Washington 16, D. C.

Folkways Records, 117 W. 46th Street, New York, New York.

Ginn and Co., Boston, Massachusetts (Auditory Training Records).

H. C. Electronics, Inc., 201 East O'Keefe, Palo Alto, California.

Linguaphone Institute, 30 Rockefeller Plaza, New York 20, New York.

Pacific Records, P.O. Box 2038D, Pasadena 2, California.

Ril Electronics Corporation, Street Road and 2nd Street Pike, Southampton, Pennsylvania.

Simon and Schuster, Rockefeller Center, New York 20, New York.

Tecnifox Corporation, Holyoke, Massachusetts.

University of California, Department of Cinema, University Park, Los Angeles 7, California.

Vicon Instrument Company, P.O. Box 2742, Colorado Springs, Colorado.

Visual Aid Materials Co., P.O. Box 66065, Los Angeles 66, California.

Jay L. Warren, Inc., 1247-49 West Belmont Avenue, Chicago 13, Illinois.

Wonderland Records, 235 W. 46th Street, New York 36, New York.

8. Evaluate the materials and equipment used during four actual therapy sessions or suggest materials a therapist could have used after you have read reports of seven of her therapy sessions.

9. Are you working with any clients who might profit from constructing some of their own therapy materials? What kind of materials? What suggestions do they have concerning materials they would like to construct?

10. Start a file of sources of materials and equipment by clipping descriptions from *ASHA's* "Clinical and Educational Materials" column. (American Speech and Hearing Association, 9030 Old Georgetown Road, Washington, D. C.)

11. Order three of the materials mentioned in the following booklet:

The Parents Volunteer Association of the Columbus State School: *Teaching Devices for Children with Impaired Learning.* 1601 West Broad Street, Columbus, Ohio, 1958.

12. A therapist made the following notes as she read the diagnostic material concerning George Adams, one of her clients for the semester. What materials would you consider appropriate for use with George?

George Adams, receptive language difficulties.

CA—nine years eight months.

Unpredictable behavior;

Immature, dependent;

Unaggravated aggressiveness, restless, short attention span;

Inability to function in a peer group;

Below-average marks in school, but average intelligence;

Enjoys books and appears to get lost in them sometimes;

Inconsistent omissions and substitutions of sounds;

Below-average grammatical structure;

Poor auditory memory span.

Chapter VII

PLANNING AND REPORTING SESSIONS

T HE WORK OF A therapist is evaluated frequently by the type
of plans and reports she writes. Good plans and reports are
written promptly, are professional, clear and appropriate.

It is important for a therapist to write plans and reports
promptly because when she delays writing them their value is
decreased and sometimes they become worthless. If she writes a
plan after the therapy session has been held, the supervisor may
give her credit for it, but his suggestions cannot help her with
the actual session. Had she been absent there would not have
been a plan for the substitute therapist ,and the therapy she
gave may have been inferior to that which she would have given
had she written the plan before she held the session.

PROFESSIONAL PLANS AND REPORTS

Skilled therapists write plans and reports that use a level of
language suited to the persons who read the reports. The plans
and reports reflect the serious, sincere and impersonal attitude
of the therapist. They are also signed and dated. When writing a
report to another speech therapist, the terminology of speech
pathology is used; however, when writing a report to parents
this terminology is not suitable.

The following reports illustrate these principles. (See Chapter
II, "Using Diagnostic Tools," for an example of a diagnostic
report.)

Summer Therapy Report

[Report was filed in the clinic and a copy was sent to the

public school therapist.]

Client: Ralph Brooks   *Therapist*: Dorothy Jones
        (mildly cerebral palsied)   *Period Covered by Report*:
Birth Date: June 25, 1952   June 29 1965, to August 6, 1965

Description of Speech at Beginning of Period

The following sounds were misarticulated: [d/g] (i), [v/ð] (m), [v/z] (f), [ʃ/tʃ] (i), (m), (f), [/dʒ] (i); [ʃ] was distorted and [l] (f) and [j] (i) were omitted. The pitch of Ralph's voice was low and monotonous, his rate monotonous and somewhat disfluent, and his quality somewhat hoarse and severely hypernasal.

Summary of Therapy

Ralph participated in direct individual speech therapy and group speech therapy sessions, each one hour in length, five days a week.

He kept a record of the number of persons with whom he talked and the number of times he was asked to repeat. He made and evaluated tape recordnigs of his voice. He discriminated between hypernasal and oral vowels and between his misarticulated consonant sounds and the acceptable production of these sounds.

The following procedures were also used:

1. Exercises to improve control of the jaw, tongue, lips and uvula;
2. Exercises to improve production of [z], [tʃ] and [dʒ];
3. Activities to encourage the use of non-nasal vowels and to increase variety in pitch during conversation.

Description of Speech at Close of the Period

Ralph had no sound substitutions, distortions, or omissions when reading and few, if any, in conversational speech. The pitch of his voice was low and monotonous and his rate was monotonous and somewhat disfluent. His vocal quality was somewhat less nasal than it was at the beginning of the period. His articulation and quality improved when he relaxed.

Impressions Concerning Client

During therapy sessions, Ralph was cooperative and mannerly. In group therapy, he was often a leader. He seemed interested in improving his speech and sometimes requested help with a particular sound; however, his attention span was relatively short.

Recommendations

Ralph does not need to attend the speech clinic program next summer, but he should have speech therapy during the school year with the public school therapist if it can be arranged.

Report to Parents

During the last six weeks, Ralph has had an individual speech lesson and a group lesson, each one hour in length, five days a week. Ralph learned to hear the mistakes he was making when pronouncing words and he learned to correct most of them. He also improved the quality of his voice. Ralph was cooperative and mannerly. He was often a leader in group therapy sessions and he seemed interested in improving his speech; however, he sometimes experienced difficulty in concentrating.

DOROTHY JONES, *Therapist*
August 6, 1965

Therapists write a more professional report when they omit first and second person pronouns, and they tend to be objective in reporting changes that have taken place in the client's speech and behavior if they administer some formal evaluations before they write the report. A therapist obtained the following information before writing a final report concerning a client with delayed speech:

Name of Test	April 30, 1964	January 1, 1965
Performance Scale of the Weschler-Intelligence Scale for Children	IQ–51	IQ–65
Illinois Test of Psycholinguistic Abilities	3 years 10 months	5 years 9 months
Mecham Developmental Language Scale	2.72 years	5.87 years

Clear Plans and Reports

Skilled therapists write plans and reports that come to the point; however, they include an adequate amount of description. The plan is so clearly written that a substitute could conduct the session in approximately the same manner.

When writing the following plan, the supervisor attempted to write clearly and to adequately describe the approach, procedures, methods, techniques, materials and equipment she planned to use. The fourteen clients who were to attend the preschool clinic had delayed speech or articulation problems.

Preschool Clinic
Plan for First Semester

September 10, 1965
Louise Clark, *Supervisor*

The objectives for the semester are:

1. To increase clients' desire to communicate;

2. To help clients organize their experiences so that they become more meaningful;

3. To improve clients' recognition and identification of the names of objects and actions;

4. To help clients form the habit of listening;

5. To improve clients' ability to articulate the sounds of American English, especially those that are easily visible and most audible.

The indirect speech therapy will be focused around units based on the following subjects: Pets and farm animals, the circus, toys and Christmas and winter fun. (Units are listed in the order of presentation.) The daily schedule is listed below:

10:00 supervised play	11:00 listening time
10:15 listening time	11:10 game time
10:25 game time	11:15 talking time
10:30 talking time	11:30 movie
10:45 tea party	

The supervisor will conduct the listening time, the tea party and during the first weeks, the game time. Later, student clinicians will conduct the game time. They will supervise the clients' play during the supervised play and they will conduct the talking time with small groups of children. The groups will be held simultaneously in various areas of the large playroom.

During the supervised play period, each client will choose where he wishes to play and his play materials. He may wish to play in the doll corner, the block corner, the game corner or at the sand table.

During the listening time, clients will bring objects from home to show and discuss, listen to stories, take part in activities and play games. Some of the stories will contain many of the easily visible and most audible sounds. Some of the stories used will be old favorites such as *The Three Bears*, while others will be more modern stories such as *Cats, Cats, Cats*. Stories and nursery rhymes will form the basis for creative play. The activities and games will present the following in play form: Ear training; vocal phonics; and production of sounds in isolation; nonsense syllables; words; phrases; and sentences.

During the game time the clients will play singing games such as "Here We Go 'Round the Mulberry Bush," simple action games such as "Going on a Lion Hunt," and finger plays.

Student clinicians will plan the therapy they will present during talking time. They will relate the therapy to the needs of the small group of clients to whom they are assigned.

Simple games or listening to phonograph records will precede the tea party. During the party, the clients will take turns passing the napkins, cookies and wastebasket. Clients will be encouraged to say "please," "thank you," etc.

Standard children's movies such as *The Little Red Hen*, will be shown at the conclusion of each day's program.

A therapst who conducted weekly direct therapy sessions with twenty high school and college-aged stutterers wrote the following plans which are based on Wendell Johnson's theory of stuttering.

Lesson Plans for Group Stuttering Therapy

First Week

OBJECTIVE: To obtain information about the clients and to encourage them to study themselves.

PROCEDURES: Clients will discuss their case histories, especially their speech histories and the theories they have as to the cause of stuttering. When necessary, the therapist will give information concerning the results of research in stuttering.

ASSIGNMENT: Keep a record of the disfluencies of normal speakers and notice how their speech and attitudes differ from the client's.

Second Week

OBJECTIVE: To convince the clients that they have the ability to talk more normally than they do.

PROCEDURES: Clients will discuss the records of the disfluencies of normal speakers. They will also discuss how the severity of their stuttering varies and under what conditions they talk more normally.

The more severe stutterers will read from a passage, omitting all words on which they expect to stutter. Clients and therapist will discuss the implications of these performances.

ASSIGNMENT: Keep a record of their actual talking time for two days.

Third Week

OBJECTIVE: To encourage the clients to analyze their speaking-time behavior.

PROCEDURES: Clients will analyze their speaking-time records. Clients will discuss the difficult situations they encountered.

ASSIGNMENT: Increase the amount of time spent in talking in easy situations.

Fourth Week

OBJECTIVE: To help each client face his problem more realistically and to reduce the number of mannerisms he has acquired.

PROCEDURES: Each client will look in a mirror as he talks and then he will describe what he has seen. He will try to eliminate his most objectionable mannerism by using negative practice and conscious control.

ASSIGNMENT: Clients will talk with individuals about their problem.

Fifth Week

OBJECTIVE: To continue to help each client face his problem.

PROCEDURES: Clients will continue mirror work while telling jokes about stutterers. Therapist will have subjects intensify the reactions that occur and will use the technique of static analysis.

ASSIGNMENT: Clients will speak in situations that are difficult for them and try to reduce the mannerisms they have acquired.

Sixth Week

OBJECTIVE: To help each client begin to modify his speech pattern.

PROCEDURES: Clients will imitate their own pattern.

ASSIGNMENT: Clients will imitate their own stuttering pattern in easy speaking situations.

Seventh Week

OBJECTIVE: To help each client modify his speech pattern.

PROCEDURES: Clients will imitate the speech patterns of others in the group during dramatizations of difficult situations.

ASSIGNMENT: Clients will imitate other speech patterns in difficult speaking situations.

Eighth Week

OBJECTIVE: To help the clients plan future therapy.

PROCEDURES: Each client will evaluate the therapy he has had and will plan future therapy.

APPROPRIATE PLANS

Good plans include an adequate number of procedures which are related to the clients' needs and are designed to reduce difficulties during therapy sessions.

Too many procedures may confuse the clients and too few may result in inefficiency. A good therapist estimates the difficulty of each procedure and allows an appropriate amount of time for each. She also provides a few more materials than she believes she will need, in case her time estimates prove inaccurate. A beginning therapist was using a therapist-constructed maze to help a young articulation client produce his sound in words. The client and therapist used the entire therapy period to complete the maze even though the client had lost interest in it. The therapist could probably have estimated the time the maze would take by seeing what part of the maze she could complete in three minutes. Then she would have shortened it before bringing it to the session. If she had not done this, she could have ended the activity during the session by saying, "We'll stop playing the game when one of us arrives at this square."

The procedures should be related to the client's needs (see Chapter III, "Using Procedures"), and designed to reduce difficulties during therapy sessions. These objectives may be partially attained by following the principals of learning. (See Chapter I, "Clinical Competence"—"Knowledge of The Learning Process.")

A supervisor once read a small random sample of daily therapy plans in order to attempt to determine how the therapists had planned to reduce difficulties during the therapy session. It seemed to the supervisor that many of the therapists had chosen materials that were related to the client's interests and abilities, in order to reduce problems. One therapist who was working with two hard-of-hearing clients had discovered that, when they played competitive games, one client was unable to accept defeat and invariably accused his opponent of cheating. She devised some materials that encouraged each client to compete with his own record and did not use competitive games.

Beginning therapists sometimes state that they do not know how to write an appropriate plan for the first therapy session. They will probably write a better plan if, before writing it, they ask themselves questions such as these about each client in the group.

What is his age, sex and speech problem?

Is his mental ability normal?

What are his interests?

Has he had speech therapy? If so, what was his attitude toward it? Why?

What can he be expected to accomplish?

After answering these questions, a therapist wrote the following plans for the first sessions with two different groups of clients:

DAILY THERAPY PLAN

BETTY LELAND
September 20, 1965

(With three college-age hypernasality clients who have not had speech therapy.)

Objectives	Procedures	Methods and/or Materials
To begin to establish a helping relationship with clients.	Obtain information from the clients.	Conversation about: favorite courses; college life; high school experiences; interests and hobbies; speech differences; speech therapy.
To begin to evaluate the current status of the problem.	Discuss speech differences and speech therapy.	
	Compare quality when reading sentences containing many nasals with quality when reading sentences that do not include nasals.	Fairbanks, G.: *Voice and Articulation Drillbook*
	Administer parts of the "Examination for Nasality."	Johnson and others: *Diagnostic Methods in Speech Correction*
	Fill out case history form.	Each client will write the information requested on the "Case History of College Client" form.

DAILY THERAPY PLAN

(With three teenaged articulation clients who have had speech therapy.)

Objectives	Procedures	Methods and/or Materials
To begin to establish helping relationships.	Converse about TV programs.	Ask questions such as: What is your favorite program? Who's your favorite star?
To begin to establish and evaluate the current status of the problem.	Tape-record a mock TV program—*What's My Line?*	Each client chooses an occupation he might like to enter. Clients take turns asking questions of each other in order to guess the occupation.
	Discuss the role of speech in the occupations chosen.	Ask questions such as: How much talking will you do if you enter this occupation? What qualities are necessary for success in the occupation?
	Play the tape recording of the mock TV program.	Each client will evaluate his own articulation by making a list of the words he thinks he has misarticulated.

If you wish to improve your ability to write professional, clear and appropriate plans and reports, the suggestions given below will help you.

Suggestions for Improving Skill in Planning and Reporting Sessions

1. Discuss with your colleagues articles similar to the following:

ENGLISH, R., AND LILLYWHITE, H.: A semantic approach to clinical reporting in speech pathology. *ASHA,* June, 1963.

2. Write a semester therapy plan for a particular group of clients. Exchange your plan with another therapist and give suggestions to each other.

3. Obtain some ideas for your next daily lesson plans from plans given in sources similar to these:

BACKUS, O., AND BEASLEY, J.: *Speech Therapy with Children.* Boston, Houghton, 1951.

BUNGER, A.: *Speech Reading, Jena Method.* Danville, Interstate Printers and Publishers.

IRWIN, R.: *Speech and Hearing Therapy.* New York, Prentice-Hall, 1953.

4. Evaluate three of the plans and reports given in this chapter.

5. Use more professional language when rewriting the following report of therapy with a university-aged client who had a hypernasal voice quality. Write a therapy plan for the client for the semester following the one reported here.

Semester Therapy Report

Working with Tom has been hit or miss. Tom missed therapy on two occasions and once through the clinician's fault, for which a new session was appointed. Therapy sessions were usually fruitful, but they were not followed up with exercise and practice. Although improvement methods were discovered they were not considered seriously enough by the client. At one time Tom discussed his problem with the supervisor. He was impressed with the possibility of his quality interfering with his success as a lawyer, but his practice fell off the following week.

Tom has said that he wants to improve his voice and also that he wishes to return to therapy. After a pep talk he said he will work more regularly. Up to this time his attitude toward therapy has been passive.

Tom enjoys school to some extent, although he often seems concerned or burdened down with work. He also has a girl friend at home whom he misses very much. He tends to be reticent and defensive at times. He often answers questions with what seem to be stock answers and he also attempts to qualify other statements that seem to reveal anything personal. He is aware of his voice problem, but he projects that it is mainly due to the tension resulting from public speaking class, and that other than that it is not much of a problem. It was explained to him, as a final stand, that unless he becomes more of an active participant in and out of therapy sessions, therapy will be fruitless.

6. Evaluate the following semester therapy play and report:

Semester Therapy Plan

Norma's problem is infantile or retarded speech. She has the following errors:

> n/l (I)
> w/l (M,F)
> ʒ/z (I,M,F)
> d/dʒ (M,F)
> t/s (I,M,F)

Distorts many blends.

Inconsistently substitutes [ʌ] for other vowels .

Norma produced [s] and [z] sounds correctly, as well as all of the vowels, upon stimulation.

GENERAL GOALS OF THERAPY

1. To establish a working relationship;
2. To evaluate speech and current status;
3. To improve client's speech;
4. Objectivity.

GENERAL METHODS OF THERAPY

1. Informal atmosphere, conversation, games and surroundings;
2. Use of various tests;
3. Material to improve articulation of sounds and production;
4. Material to improve self-concept and self-realization.

Report of Therapy

Norma can produce the [s] correctly in words, sentences

and conversation most of the time. She uses correct [ʃ] and [l] sounds in isolated words, the [ʃ] being the better of the two and extending into correct production in conversation in most cases. She talks at a slower rate and has acquired skill in evaluation of her own speech.

7. Compare the daily therapy plans and reports presented below. They were written by two therapists who were helping the same nine-year-old functional articulation client during two different semesters.

Plan I

Procedures	Methods and/or Materials	Report
1. Review of sound production.	Materials from the clinic.	The client is making progress.
2. Practice the sound in stories.		

Plan II

Procedures	Methods and/or Materials	Report
1. Use sound matching techniques.	Van Riper: *Speech Correction: Principles and Methods.*	Jim responded very well and corrected himself whenever he made errors. He was enthusi-
2. Take tongue exercises.	*Tony Plays with Sounds.*	astic with the tongue exercises and did them after he was
3. Participate in sound isolation techniques.	Read story and poem from *Tony Plays with Sounds.* Review last assignments. Think of words that contain his sound in I, M, and F positions.	told to stop. He says the sound well in isolation, but because he speaks so fast he leaves off endings and tends to slur them. The tape recording went well. He was anxious to hear how he
4. Reduce speaking rate.	Use tape recorder and negative practice, breath control exercises.	sounded and when he heard how fast he sounded he put his hands over his ears. He needs much work in slowing down his speech and drill on the [s] in F position.

8. A therapist who was giving therapy to a college-aged client with a hoarse voice rewrote the following daily therapy plan after a conference with her supervisor. In what respects is the revision superior to the original plan? What changes would you make in the revision?

Original Plan

OBJECTIVES: To make Emma aware of her voice;

To relax her vocal cords;

To try to find a more suitable pitch.

PROCEDURES: Record free speech and oral reading;
Speak in whispers and with breathiness;
Use different ranges and evaluate in terms of sound and tension.

Revised Plan

OBJECTIVES: To increase Emma's awareness of her pitch, range intensity and quality;
To increase Emma's awareness of the sound of her voice and possible variations.

PROCEDURES: 1. Read and record a short passage:
Using habitual pitch level;
Using a higher pitch level;
Using a lower pitch level;
Using a greater loudness level;
Using a softer loudness level.
2. Record sustained vowels varying the pitch, intensity and rate;
3. Record paired word lists;
4. Record conversational speech varying the pitch, intensity and rate.

9. Therapists frequently modify their plans during actual therapy sessions. Evaluate the changes that a therapist made when giving therapy to a severe stutterer who was ten years old.

Plan I

1. Informal conversation about herself and her speech;
2. Successive reading of a passage to test adaptation.

Report of Session I

Sally stuttered severely when talking about herself and her speech. At times the therapist could not understand her. Stopped the conversation and played a game that required no speech. Eventually Sally started talking about the game and her speech was more fluent. Sally drew pictures of the members of her family instead of reading the passage and talked some as she made the drawings. She wrote a short paragraph describing how she feels when she stutters.

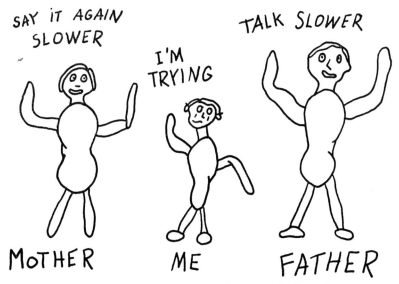

Drawn by a ten-year-old stutterer when she was asked to draw a picture of herself and her parents when she was stuttering. She later remarked, "I hope they never see that picture of me crying."

Plan II

1. Explain prolongation;
2. Therapist and client read a poem and prolong the initial sounds;
3. Tape-record a mock interview.

Report of Session II

Sally would not read using prolongation. She said that she never wanted to hear anyone read that way again. Choral reading was used, omitting the prolongation. She was disappointed that she was not going to play a game. A sentence constructing game was devised and I showed her how we could play a game and work on her speech at the same time. She talked about some friends who had teased her about her speech. She stuttered severely when attempting to tape the interview and so we used role-playing to illustrate ways of reacting to teasing.

10. Write a semester plan for language therapy for the client whose therapy report is presented below.

Client: Clarence Stevens—
    Delayed Speech   January, 1966
Period of Therapy: October 1965 to   *Student Clinician—*
            January 1966   Ellis James

Summary of Therapy

Indirect therapy was used with Clarence during most of the sessions held this semester, because he was unwilling to communicate and the therapy period seemed to threaten him. The clinician avoided correcting his articulation and language and listened attentively to any remarks he made. He was encouraged to use the words he understood. His desire and ability to communicate verbally improved. During the last weeks of therapy the clinician began direct therapy on the identification of colors. At the last session Clarence identified red and yellow.

RESULTS OF THE ILLINOIS TEST OF PSYCHOLINGUISTIC ABILITIES

On November 16, when Clarence was five years two months old, the above test was administered to him. The results were as follows:

	Language Age
Auditory Vocal Automatic Test	5-4
(test of grammar)	
Auditory Vocal Association	4-11
(answers to questions, such as, "I sit in a chair, I sleep on a ?")	
Vocal Encoding	4-1
(describing common objects)	
Audiotry Vocal Sequencing	3-9
(repeating series of digits)	
Auditory Decoding	2-9
(answers questions such as "Do dogs bark?")	

The validity of the Auditory Decoding Subtest was questioned because Clarence nodded his head in response to every question; however, he appeared to understand the directions before the test was administered. During the administration of some of the other subtests, some perseveration was noticed and often he seemed to need to repeat what was said to him in order to retain it.

RECOMMENDATIONS

1. Continued speech and language therapy at the Speech Clinic;

2. Conference with the parents to point out the possible consequences of undue pressure for acceptable speech from Clarence. Conference conducted by the Supervisor of clinicians at the Speech Clinic.

Chapter VIII

EVALUATING THERAPY

A<small>UTHORITIES</small> <small>FREQUENTLY</small> emphasize the importance of a client, especially an older one, becoming skilled in evaluating his own speech and in improving his ability to modify it without help from a therapist. It also seems important for a therapist to improve her skill in evaluating therapy in order to improve it. A therapist improves her ability to evaluate therapy by becoming more objective, increasing insight into her own strengths and limitations and developing a desire to improve.

Some therapists spend too much time evaluating therapy and they are too critical of the therapy they administer. Others seldom evaluate themselves as therapists and seldom criticize their therapy. Both types of therapists should become more skilled in evaluating therapy.

A SKILLED THERAPIST IS OBJECTIVE

It is, perhaps, impossible for a therapist to become entirely objective when evaluating the therapy she administers; however, she should attempt frequently to view therapy in an impartial manner.

Sometimes she becomes more objective by asking herself questions similar to the following:

> How is the client getting along in therapy?
> Is his speech improving?
> What can I do to help him improve faster?
> If the client continues to improve at the present rate, will he have improved enough by the close of the semester

for me to recommend that he be dismissed? Should I expect him to make this much improvement? Why, or why not?

A beginning therapist wrote the following weekly evaluations of therapy with a nine-year-old client who had an expressive language problem:

> Gerald enjoyed the therapy session and worked hard. The materials provided held his interest. He still does not realize, however, that he can improve his speech by using a slower rate.
>
> Gerald was very restless during the first part of the session. He soon lost interest in listening to a tape recording of his reading and should have been provided with a shorter story to record and some activity that would have encouraged discriminative listening. He talked freely as he placed the farm animals on the felt board, but his sentence structure was poor.
>
> Gerald's articulation seemed to improve following a careful explanation of how he was misarticulating the words of a drill. Too much time was spent in making a speech notebook and there was no time for role playing. Activities should have been provided that would have helped to decrease his restlessness.

A SKILLED THERAPIST HAS INSIGHT

A skilled therapist has insight into her own strengths and limitations. As she becomes more objective her insight increases.

A therapist who has difficulty developing her ability to evaluate her strengths and limitations may obtain help from clients, supervisors, colleagues and parents of clients. She may ask older clients for oral or written evaluations, using adaptations of evaluation forms employed by classroom teachers, or she may ask clients to write a paragraph, evaluating the therapy they are receiving. She may ask a younger client to conduct a therapy session and she will often discover that he is conducting the session in much the same manner that she has been using. Supervisors, colleagues and parents may also help evaluate therapy, but the therapist remains the prime evaluator.

After careful self-study and after obtaining evaluations from others, a therapist used the Clinical Competence Form given in Chapter I to help her write the following evaluation of her therapy:

I am usually aware of the client's defective sound productions and I understand much about the way in which sounds are produced. I am acquainted with many of the currently accepted therapeutic procedures used with the type of problems my clients have. I believe that I understand some of the feelings and the individual aspects of at least a few of my clients.

I generally use procedures that are related to the client's problem and that are challenging. I explain methods and techniques clearly and I use a variety of materials. My plans and reports are prompt and clear.

I should improve my knowledge of the factors that are related to clients' organic problems and I need to have a better understanding of the theories of learning and to apply one theory more consistently.

I am skilled in creating a warm friendly atmosphere with a small group of shy clients, but with a larger group of young active clients I need to be more firm and a better disciplinarian.

I try to be objective when evaluating therapy, but I have a tendency to let others' remarks influence me too much. If someone is critical of a method I have used I am hurt and can not adequately evaluate the results of the method.

Some therapists need to evaluate their communication skills. Several need to improve their eye contact with listeners, some need to improve their use of grammar and some should use more effective gestures. Some are mild clutterers and/or need to improve their vocal pitch, quality or articulation. One male therapist had a higher pitch level than his client, whose problem was a high pitch level. Another therapist used a different quality when talking with a mentally retarded client than she used with her other clients. Another needed to improve her production of some vowels.

A SKILLED THERAPIST DESIRES TO IMPROVE

The evaluations that a therapist makes have little value unless she tries to improve. After she determines her limitations she should try to eliminate some of them or at least weaken them. She should build up new habits to take the place of the old and realize that self-study and learning are difficult procedures, but not necessarily uninteresting, for both therapists and clients.

Suggestions for Improving Skill in Evaluating Therapy

1. How much time do you spend in evaluating therapy? Should you increase or decrease the amount of time spent?

2. Write an evaluation of your therapy with the client (or group of clients) making the least progress in speech improvement.

3. Make a tape recording of one of your therapy sessions with a preschool client. Diagnose your own speech. What should you do first to improve your voice, articulation or language?

4. After reading the following article, measure the "Therapist-Client Interaction" by making a judgment every ten seconds as you play the tape recording mentioned in suggestion 4:

MERRILL, B.: A measurement of mother-child interaction. *J Abnor Soc Psychol, 41*:37-49, 1946.

How can you improve the interaction? Discuss the results of your measurement with your supervisor and/or your colleagues.

5. Ask a client to write a description of a therapy session. While he is writing it you write one too. Compare the descriptions.

6. Adapt an evaluation form used by classroom teachers, in order to make it more appropriate as an evaluation form of speech therapy. Ask older clients to use the form to evaluate the therapy you administer.

7. Discuss the progress one of your clients is making in therapy with his parents.

8. Creativity may be defined as the ability to discover a unique solutoin to a problem. Describe the major problem of one of your clients and think of two solutions that might be considered unique. Evaluate the solutions and try the one you consider the better of the two. Evaluate the results.

9. Construct a graph on which you may plot the weekly changes that one of your older clients makes in one aspect of his speech, language or behavior. Ask the client to make a similar graph or to develop his own method of evaluating his progress.

Compare the graphs or records at regular intervals.

10. Compare the following evaluations of therapy with articulation clients:

Client I

There is no problem eliciting speech from Jim. He speaks to the clinician with ease and there is an overall free atmosphere of speech. Jim seems very conscious of the "s" problem and tries very hard to say it the new way. The only time he slips is on the blends. Therefore, much time should be spent on drill words containing the blends. Jim will add to his problem list every session.

Client II

Keith is willing to participate in speech activities, but it seems evident that he will not be able to do much abstract thinking in therapy. The materials used will have to be concrete as it seems difficult for him to concentrate. He is capable of being involved in simple activities, with but one or two necessary directions. He tires out easily. The therapist had to point out to him that there will be things she'll let him do and other things he'll be asked not to do. Conversation helps the therapist determine which sounds are being carried-over. Drawing faces on the blackboard appeals to Keith and helps the therapist illustrate points she wishes to get across to him. He can distinguish voiced from voiceless sounds, but he needs further explanation of what happens to make a sound voiced.

11. What are some procedures that the therapist who wrote the following evaluation might follow in order to improve her therapy sessions?

The therapist should have been more familar with the articulation test she attempted to administer. She included too many activities in the therapy plan. Taking more time for an activity helped Jim see the purpose in the activity and gave him a chance to accomplish more. Jim's writing ability was underestimated. He's using cursive writing rather than printing. The therapist should have been more organized.

She should make therapy more enjoyable and give Jim more rewards.

12. After discussing the following article with a group of therapists, apply the technique to some of the first therapy sessions you have with a stutterer:

MATHEWSON, R., AND ROCHLIN, L.: Analysis of unstructured self-appraisal; a technique in counselor-education. *J Counsel Psychol, 3*:22-36.

13. Compile a list of your limitations as a therapist. Add to the list after obtaining some opinions from clients. You may wish to ask older clients to write an evaluation of one therapy session or have the members of a group of younger clients take turns teaching the group. Which client seemed to imitate you most accurately? Have other young clients draw pictures of you or of "What We Do in Speech Class," "How I Feel Today," "What I Like About Coming Here" or "What I Don't Like Here."

Which of your limitations do you believe should be corrected first? List three steps you plan to take in order to improve this aspect of your behavior.

14. After consulting sources similar to the following, compare the evaluation of public school speech therapy with the evaluation of classroom teaching in the elementary school:

IRWIN, R.: *Speech and Hearing Therapy.* Englewood Cliffs, Prentice-Hall, 1953, pp. 204-205.

KNIGHT, P.: *Qualities Related to Success in Teaching.* New York, Teachers College, Columbia.

LINDSAY, M., MOUTH, L., AND GROTBERG, E.: *Improving Laboratory Experiences in Teacher Education.* New York, Teachers College, Columbia, pp. 131-141.

MEDLEY, D., AND KLEIN, A.: Measuring classroom behavior with a pupil-reaction inventory. *Elementary School J., 57*:315-319, Mar., 1957.

MONROE, W., AND CLARK, J.: *Measuring Teaching Efficiency.* Urbana, U of Ill.

RUGG, H.: *A Rating Scale for Judging Teachers in Service.* Chicago, U of Chicago.

RYANS, D.: *Characteristics of Teachers.* Washington, D. C., ACE, 1960.

The Wilson teacher-appraisal scale. Chicago, Administrative Research Associates, Box 1160.

15. After reading from sources similar to the following, discuss with a group of colleagues some of the personal emotional factors which may be limiting your success as a therapist:

JERSILD, A.: *When Teachers Face Themselves*. New York, Teachers College, Columbia, 1955.

NAME INDEX

SUBJECT INDEX

A

American Speech and Hearing
   Association:
   conventions of, 21-22
   cumulative indexes of the journals
      of, 91
Aphasia:
   aspects of, 16-17
   diagnosis, 26-32, 43
   films concerning, 43, 70
   screening evaluations of, 35
   tests for, 38-39
Aphasia, therapy for:
   film concerning, 70
   methods of, 88
   objectives of, 31-32, 69, 74
   procedures of, 74
Articulation:
   film concerning, 10
   increasing knowledge of, 12
   interests of client, 16
   testing of, 35-37
Articulation, therapy for:
   daily plans and reports, 119, 122
   ear training in, 82-83
   evaluation of, 130-131
   grouping in, 72-73
   learning in, 18-19
   materials of, 97-100
   methods of, 79-81, 84-87, 89-90
   objectives of, 65, 67-69, 75-76
   phonetics in, 7-10
   procedures of, 65, 67-69, 75-76
   reflection of feelings in, 48-49
   selection of sounds, 66-67, 72
   semester plan of, 114-115
   transcript of session, 51-52

*Articulatory Movements in the
   Production of English Speech
   Sounds* (a film), 10
ASHA, 110
Atmosphere, creating an:
   by helpful therapists, 50-54
   by self-confident therapists, 56-57
   by understanding therapists, 46-50
   suggestions for improving skill in,
      57-63
Attitudes:
   methods for improving, 77-80
   of a delayed speech client, 32
   of cerebral palsied client, 16
   of stutterers, 32-33, 78
   of therapists, 46-57
   understanding of, 16
*Auditorially Handicapped Child,
   The* (a film), 43
Auditory factors:
   diagnosis of, 41, 43
   ear training, 18, 82-83, 97

B

Basic Audiometric Testing (a film), 43
Behavior:
   observation of, 40
   problems of, 15-16, 17
   Also see Atmosphere, creating an

C

Case history:
   abstracting of, 13
   forms for, 40
   of aphasia client, 30-31